PRAISE FOR *CHANGING CHILDREN'S LIVES WITH HYPNOSIS*

"Mainstream medicine too often focuses on drugs and gadgets at the expense of health fundamentals. Dr. Ran D. Anbar makes a compelling case for using hypnosis to leverage the mind-body connection and, in many cases, empower patients to heal themselves. Everyone should read this book to understand how hypnosis can be a powerfully effective instrument for diagnosis, treatment, and more, and why it should become as common a tool in health care as a stethoscope or prescription pad."
—**Hy Bender**, *New York Times*–bestselling author of over twenty books, including *Take Charge of Your Thyroid Disorder*

"In *Changing Children's Lives with Hypnosis*, Dr. Anbar has taken the medical/clinical topic of hypnosis, which has long been looked upon with confusion and skepticism, and woven it into relatable, readable, gripping, heart-warming—and occasionally heart-wrenching—stories that shine light on this underutilized field of medicine. Dr. Anbar was my first professor of clinical hypnosis fifteen years ago, transforming my pediatric pulmonology and sleep medicine practice (and my life) completely through his extensive expertise and indefatigable mentorship. Learning from Dr. Anbar has always been awe-inspiring. Readers of *Changing Children's Lives with Hypnosis* will soon know why."
—**Lewis J. Kass**, MD, FAAP, director of pediatric sleep medicine, Norwalk Hospital Westchester Pediatric Pulmonology and Sleep Medicine, Westchester Center for Clinical Hypnosis

"Dr. Anbar is a renowned leader in the field of mind-body medicine and medical hypnosis. This book will help open people's eyes to the power we each possess for self-regulation. Readers, especially parents, will appreciate learning how suggestions and mental imagery may be used to influence conditions as diverse as anxiety, pain, asthma, insomnia, low self-esteem, and bedwetting." —**D. Corydon Hammond**, PhD, author of *Handbook of Hypnotic Suggestion and Metaphors*, professor emeritus at University of Utah School of Medicine, past president of American Society of Clinical Hypnosis

"Plato said that the mind and the body are one and should not be treated separately. The compelling stories in this book are in that tradition and illustrate how self-hypnosis can be a tool to help children take control over disruptive symptoms." —**Drucy Borowitz**, MD, emeritus clinical professor of pediatrics, Jacobs School of Medicine and Biomedical Sciences, Buffalo, New York

"Dr. Anbar's commitment to helping his pediatric patients is evident throughout his new book, *Changing Children's Lives with Hypnosis*. You don't need be a doctor to appreciate his winning ways; he explains his methods in an easy-to-understand format, and the reader gets to observe the entire, fascinating process. Please read this book if you know a child who is suffering—you may be able to steer the family toward relief." —**Roberta Temes**, PhD, author of *The Complete Idiot's Guide to Hypnosis*, faculty (retired) Downstate Medical School, Brooklyn, New York

"Over the past twenty years Dr. Anbar has embarked on an intense study of hypnosis through countless workshops, persistent inquiries, writing, and careful listening to colleagues, mentors, and, most of all, his young patients. *Changing Children's Lives with Hypnosis*, with its stories that variably astound, challenge, and inspire, is an important and courageous undertaking. Through his clear commitment to the power of language and the human mind to create change, Dr. Anbar teaches young people, their families, and their clinicians to believe that positive change is both possible and doable." —**Daniel P. Kohen**, MD, FAAP, ABMH Developmental-Behavioral Pediatrics, Kohen Therapy Associates; director of developmental-behavioral pediatrics program and professor, Departments of Pediatrics and Family Medicine and

Community Health, University of Minnesota (retired); cofounder and director of education, National Pediatric Hypnosis Training Institute; coauthor of *Hypnosis and Hypnotherapy with Children*

"*Changing Children's Lives with Hypnosis* is a wonderful new addition to the literature on clinical hypnosis with children. Dr. Anbar is a top expert in this field. His clinical experience in pediatric medicine and children's mental health enables him to bring this valuable information and hypnotic approaches with children to other professionals in the field. Highly recommended!" —**William C. Wester II**, EdD, retired psychologist, past president of the American Society of Clinical Hypnosis

"I was always a cynic when 'hypnosis' was suggested as a medical alternative. But then, thirty years ago, I became the father of a profoundly physically challenged young boy—a quadriplegic child, dependent on a ventilator. He was 'locked in' by his condition, and nothing was available to open the window to his heart and soul. Then along came Dr. Anbar, a highly respected pediatric pulmonologist, who told me, 'I think I can help!' There were no hollow pronouncements, just 'I think, through good medicine and the introduction of hypnosis, we can improve the quality of your son's life.' And he did. This book is not an esoteric medical manuscript, but rather a book about life and for life. Dr. Anbar and his story exemplify wisdom, determination, passion, creativity, and willingness to 'go the extra mile' for the children in his care." —**Rabbi Charles S. Sherman**, MBIEE-Melrose B'nai Israel Emanu-El, author of *The Broken and the Whole*

"I believe that hypnosis is one of the more powerful tools available to medicine. Dr. Anbar's book is a great way to learn about this powerful tool. In formal hypnosis, we engage the patient to help him or her learn to utilize self-hypnosis. But words have incredible power, and our choice of words, augmented by tone of voice, body language, and the like, can often have the same effect as they might in a formal session of 'hypnosis.' I highly recommend Dr. Anbar's book. The concepts he discusses are useful to medical practitioners and also to parents (and even grandparents). Suggestion is powerful. It can be positive or negative, deliberate or inadvertent. This book will help the reader become more aware of the power of our words and lower the chances of our using inadvertent negative suggestion, with undesired consequences." —**Robert E. Wood**, PhD, MD, emeritus professor, pediatrics and otolaryngology, division of pulmonary medicine, Cincinnati Children's Hospital

"I have known Dr. Anbar for over twenty-five years through his affiliation as a local and national medical advisor for Make-A-Wish. I witnessed a colleague's four-year old daughter completely replace sedation with self-hypnosis for her MRIs as follow-up for brain tumor treatment. As a lay person, I have long admired Dr. Anbar as a true champion for children's health care. His compassion and willingness to listen to and validate what his patients tell him is genuine and central to patient care. This, coupled with his out-of-the-box approach on how best to serve his patients, has helped thousands of children live healthier, happier, more hopeful lives." —**Diane E. Kuppermann**, Syracuse, New York

"In this powerful book, Dr. Anbar brings his deep and broad clinical experience to show us how he has helped young people with a variety of profound health challenges use their imaginative capacity to enrich their lives. Through these very personal and even intimate windows, he gives us a vision of how using hypnosis to carefully empower people seeking health care can revolutionize health and care." —**Laurence Irwin Sugarman**, MD, FAAP, ABMH, College of Health Sciences and Technology, Rochester Institute of Technology

Changing Children's Lives with Hypnosis

Changing Children's Lives with Hypnosis

A Journey to the Center

RAN D. ANBAR, MD

ROWMAN & LITTLEFIELD
Lanham • Boulder • New York • London

Published by Rowman & Littlefield
An imprint of The Rowman & Littlefield Publishing Group, Inc.
4501 Forbes Boulevard, Suite 200, Lanham, Maryland 20706
www.rowman.com

86-90 Paul Street, London EC2A 4NE, United Kingdom

British Library Cataloguing in Publication Information Available

Library of Congress Cataloging-in-Publication Data

The previous edition was catalogued by the Library of Congress as follows:

Names: Anbar, Ran D., author.
Title: Changing children's lives with hypnosis : a journey to the center / Ran D. Anbar, MD.
Description: Lanham : Rowman & Littlefield Publishers, 2021. | Includes bibliographical references and index. | Summary: "Hypnosis is a grossly underused tool in pediatric medicine to address both physical and psychological symptoms. This technique helps manage anxiety, breathing issues, habits, pain, and countless other concerns. The book unfolds as a pediatrician recognizes the healing power of hypnosis and offers families ways to incorporate aspects of hypnosis at home"— Provided by publisher.
Subjects: LCSH: Hypnotism—Therapeutic use. | Child psychotherapy.
Classification: LCC RJ505.H86 A53 2021 (print) | LCC RJ505.H86 (ebook) | DDC 615.8/512083—dc23
LC record available at https://lccn.loc.gov/2021020054
LC ebook record available at https://lccn.loc.gov/2021020055

ISBN: 978-1-5381-5366-6 (cloth)
ISBN: 978-1-5381-8547-6 (pbk)
ISBN: 978-1-5381-5367-3 (ebook)

To Paul, my patient, mentor, guide, and friend.

Your curiosity about a little-known medical intervention, your natural ability to use it, and your openness to new adventures helped introduce me to the rich world of hypnosis and the healing power it holds. It is my privilege to carry on this work we started together.

Contents

Acknowledgments

I would like to thank the many people who helped shape this book. First and foremost, I thank Jana Murphy, my writing partner, who helped organize the patient stories in this book in a way that effectively and eloquently builds an understanding of my experiences with hypnosis. Through our work together, I learned that Jana puts her heart and soul into her writing, and thus she and I share a passion for our respective vocations.

I also want to acknowledge my wife, Hannah, who has supported the development of my hypnosis practice over the past two decades and the writing of this book. I very much appreciate that Hannah served as my first editor for all of the drafts of this book. It's funny to think back to when I first encountered and became excited about hypnosis, a time when Hannah expressed concern about whether I might end up as a guru on top of a mountain. I'm happy to report that instead of retreating to a mountain, I've been working to bring hypnosis into the mainstream in the valley with Hannah by my side.

I am fortunate to have had the opportunity to share drafts of the book with readers who've given me invaluable feedback that helped make it better. These readers include Rohan Achar, my son Dr. Joshua Anbar, Dr. Danielle Aretz, Dr. Cheryl Beighle, Christopher Costello, Pastor Nancy Duff, Dr. Steven Eisenberg, Sherrie Jacoby, Dr. Lewis

Kass, Dr. Robert Kellman, Jeff Lipton, Dr. Nadia Sarwar, Dr. Moshe Torem, and Dr. Joseph Zastrow. I am very grateful to my agent, Alice Martell, for her enthusiastic support and steadfast commitment to finding a good home for the book, and my editor at Rowman & Littlefield, Suzanne Staszak-Silva, who has encouraged me along the way. Thanks also to Beth Easter, Jen Kelland, Diana Nuhn, Deni Remsberg, Jennifer Rushing-Schurr, Patricia Stevenson, and the other R&L team members who've helped guide this book to publication.

I want to especially acknowledge and sincerely thank my patients for teaching me much of what I learned about hypnosis and especially about the subconscious. Working with you challenges and inspires me, constantly opens my eyes to new possibilities, and brings joy and fulfillment to my life.

Introduction

In a world with a seemingly endless array of medical and pharmaceutical interventions available for nearly any health issue, why consider hypnosis?

It's a fair question, and as a physician with a specialized background in pediatric pulmonary disorders, there was a time when I asked it myself.

The simple answer is that treatment using hypnosis works. It's been more than twenty years since I started offering this therapy to my patients—initially motivated to explore it by a teenage boy with a life-threatening diagnosis who was clearly not getting everything he needed from the standard medical protocols. Since then, I've found that nearly every child with chronic illness and/or mental health challenges can benefit from a combination of hypnosis and counseling.

Some improvements are essential pieces of a much larger puzzle—increased confidence, improved concentration, better sleep, overcoming phobias, and the ability to create distance from pain or anxiety. Some engage extraordinary shifts—patients who overcome maladies that kept them from going to school, from making friends, from living normal lives; patients who might otherwise be hospitalized or institutionalized if not for the changes therapeutic hypnosis brought them.

The reason hypnosis benefits children with a broad range of symptoms is in part that its use for therapy is unique in meeting them where they have the most need. In many children with chronic illness, for example, the burden of their medical issues leads to anxiety, depression, or other psychological reactions. By learning how to use hypnosis to better regulate themselves emotionally, these children can handle their illnesses with less psychological distress and more resilience. In children whose psychological burdens cause them to develop physical symptoms, those symptoms often resolve completely when the children learn to understand and regulate their feelings and responses. Finally, almost every child can benefit from learning how to control their negative reactions to uncomfortable medical procedures and stressful situations.

The impacts of these improvements change children's lives, and the resulting ripples alter the lives of their families as well. Kids use the tools they learn in hypnosis to get on with schooling, activities, and sports, to plan for their futures, and to enjoy day-to-day pleasures that were once lost to them. They feel better, and they feel better about themselves as they learn how to employ self-empowerment. Parents are sometimes able to relinquish the constant and crushing worry about whether a sick or troubled child is going to be okay. Often siblings are able to begin stepping out of the shadows of brothers and sisters who've required the lion's share of the family's attention. Taken as a whole, these changes have a profound influence on how families function.

Incorporating hypnosis into my own medical practice began slowly, but within a year I was offering it to dozens of patients, and then to hundreds. As my interest in it and success grew, I opened my practice to general pediatric patients in addition to those dealing with lung problems. Pediatricians began referring kids they thought might benefit from hypnosis, as well as patients with whom they'd hit diagnostic walls. When those patients improved (often quickly), referrals flooded in. I started working Sundays to accommodate patients I didn't have time to see during the week.

At the outset of this journey, I had no idea that within a few years I'd realize I could accomplish more healing every day, week, month, and year with hypnosis than I could through traditional medicine alone. With that understanding at heart, I founded a hypnosis-centered practice. Today, I see patients with a wide range of medical and psychological problems, and I train other physicians and health care providers to provide hypnosis therapy.

Every day I see patients taking steps—sometimes tentative baby steps and sometimes giant leaps—toward wellness and self-determination. I see kids who feel more in control of their own well-being than they once thought possible. Their breakthroughs and progress are the reasons I can't wait to get up each morning and can't wait to get to work.

This book is organized to help you learn about the possibilities and intricacies of hypnosis therapy in the same gradual way I experienced it: first, by focusing on what hypnosis is and how it works; second, by delving into the power of words to create feelings and images and the way those creations drive successful therapy; third, by looking more deeply into the unique access hypnosis offers to the subconscious and how its power can be harnessed by both patient and therapist; and last, by exploring the social and spiritual implications of this treatment that go beyond addressing and resolving physical and psychological symptoms.

Throughout this book, I've included suggestions that parents, caregivers, teachers, and medical professionals can use to incorporate the empowering tools of hypnotic technique into everyday life. You'll also find at the end of the book two chapters dedicated to hypnosis-inspired steps families can take on their own. Although there is no substitute for the level of hypnosis therapy a trained medical provider can offer, there are many ways families can incorporate the logic of its concepts into their interactions and relationships.

My experience amounts to a mountain of anecdotal evidence that hypnosis therapy works, and there is a growing body of scientific evidence to match. The fact is that medical and counseling professionals

at all levels would benefit from training in this mode of therapy—and
their pediatric patients, in turn, would benefit from its incorporation
as a first-line treatment option. Until there's enough demand for that
training (which requires a miniscule time commitment compared to the
rigors of medical school or a graduate program in psychology), patients
won't routinely be given this option. Many won't even know it exists. If
you as a parent are given hope or even curiosity about hypnosis therapy
after reading this book, I urge you to ask your child's doctors about it.
Ultimately, patient demand can bring this gentle, effective healing tool
into the mainstream, where it belongs.

In many cultures and religions, our spiritual center is thought to be
the inner place where we achieve physical, mental, and emotional peace.
Reaching this positive, productive, hopeful state of mind is a goal we
naturally gravitate toward, even when we're not thinking about it. My
experience with hypnosis therapy has allowed me the privilege of helping countless children find this space and learn to visit it at will. My
hope is that this book helps lead many more children to navigate their
own journey to the center.

I

THE POWER OF HYPNOSIS

The Deep, Clear Lake

More Questions Than Answers

Breathing is essential to life, but most of us spend our days and nights oblivious to it, blessed with healthy, functioning lungs that work for us on autopilot.

As a pediatric pulmonologist, I've often treated patients who can't take that simplest of human necessities—inhaling and filling their lungs with oxygen—for granted. For myriad reasons, their lungs sometimes fail, leaving them gasping, wheezing, or, in the severest cases, tethered to ventilators that provide each breath.

To the untrained eye, most of my pulmonology patients, even those with the most serious respiratory issues, look just like other kids. They act like them too: they laugh, play, pout, and rebel. But because they have asthma, cystic fibrosis (CF), or other pulmonary conditions, they almost universally have experienced significant challenges in their lives and know what it's like to struggle for air.

I've had the privilege of working with thousands of patients over my career, and many of them have made lasting impressions on me. Two of them in particular, however, I remember not just for their unique medical circumstances and the bond we shared but also because it's fair to say each changed the course of my life. Each of them was integral to the path that brought me to understand that therapy with hypnosis is an invaluable tool for children's health and well-being.

THE UNACCEPTABLE DISEASE

I was sixteen years old and volunteering in a California children's hospital's child life program in the 1970s when I met the first of these patients, a boy named Harry. My task was to interact with the kids, to help take their minds off their medical conditions and treatments and the fact that they were stuck in the hospital. On my first day, I scanned the playroom looking for someone to engage, and there was Harry, leaning against a wall, one hand propped on an IV pole from which a suspended opaque bag steadily dripped fluid into his arm. He looked to be eight or nine years old, alert and interested in the different exchanges going on around him. I introduced myself, chatted a few minutes, and asked about his IV.

"It's my treatment. IV drugs for two weeks; then I can go home. Cystic fibrosis," he sighed. "I have to be here a lot."

I asked whether Harry might like to do something together, thinking maybe we'd play checkers or cards, but he had a bolder idea.

"Let's play football!"

I glanced over at the program director, wondering if such a physical game was a good idea, but it quickly became clear Harry had done this before. He opened an equipment closet, grabbed a ball, and led the way to the door—all the while steering the IV pole, which seemed so cumbersome to me, as if it were a natural appendage.

Outside on a small lawn, we tossed the ball back and forth. Harry seemed more at ease in the sunshine, and while we played, we chatted about his friends and the upcoming school year.

I lobbed the ball his way and asked what grade.

"Seventh!" he said.

Hang on. I looked at the boy again. Was he a prodigy? Or was he much older than he appeared?

"I'm twelve," Harry smiled, reading my mind. It wasn't until much later I'd learn that slowed growth is typical of many patients with CF, but Harry's revelation about his age went a long way toward explaining why this seemingly little boy was so funny and relatable to my not-much-older self.

Over the next two weeks, when we weren't tossing a football between us, Harry and I played countless hands of rummy, hours of checkers, and a couple of epic Monopoly games. One evening, after the playroom closed, I asked the therapy supervisor about Harry's condition, mentioning how remarkably upbeat he was for a kid who was so often stuck in the hospital.

"He may think of this place almost like a second home," she explained. "Kids can adapt to a lot of less-than-ideal circumstances. Harry spends so much time here, he's learned to make the best of it."

I nodded and then opened a line of inquiry that had been worrying me for days, ever since I'd read that cystic fibrosis was a fatal disease. "Harry doesn't look that sick," I said, not daring to ask a direct question about the expected length of his life.

"It's true," she agreed, "and right now he doesn't feel that sick. But his disease is rapidly progressive."

I asked how rapid. I was afraid to hear the answer but felt this was something I had a responsibility to understand.

"Most kids with CF as severe as Harry's live into their late teens."

My stomach dropped. I'd hoped what I'd been reading was wrong. Late teens is just the beginning of a life.

After a quiet minute, I asked the only other question I could think of: "Is there anything I can do for him?"

"Yes, there is," she said. "You can help make Harry's time in the hospital more enjoyable."

I could definitely do that. I was already thinking of Harry as a friend, not just a kid I played checkers with for the program. When he went home and I went back to school, we agreed to be pen pals, and for years afterward we exchanged letters about our favorite books, movies, jokes, and what was going on in our lives.

Once in a while, we'd get together in person. Harry visited me in Chicago while I was in medical school, and we went to a Cubs game together. I also went to see him in California to admire and celebrate his newly minted driver's license. Harry grinned widely as he adjusted his mirrors, seats, and sunglasses multiple times, and then he proceeded to drive me around town. That's how I remember him: a small, smart, proud young man in aviators, cracking me up from the driver's seat as we talked about the life goals that come after driving.

Harry would not get to achieve most of his goals. Each time I saw him, he was thinner and his cough was worse. As my medical training progressed, it opened my eyes to the extent that the fight against CF can be a losing battle.

It was a starkly cold January morning in Chicago when Harry's mom called to tell me he'd passed away, surrounded by his family. He was nineteen. We'd been pen pals and then friends for seven years. Like most kids born with CF during that time, Harry could never reasonably expect to have the kind of future most people take for granted: a job, a family, and an independent adult life. If he'd been born thirty years later, he would have been able to take the groundbreaking medications that now allow CF patients to live much longer, fuller lives.

Instead, he became one of the many children who inspired scientists and doctors to find a better way to care for those patients.

My friendship with Harry and witnessing his suffering helped me reach two consequential realizations. First, I wanted to be a part of the field that would one day cure CF. The disease was unacceptable— senseless and cruel, with frustrating treatment options that weren't nearly enough. We had to be able to do better, and Harry's fate was one of the most compelling reasons for me to choose pediatric pulmonary medicine as my specialty. Second, I saw firsthand that chronic illness requires more than just medical treatment. Physical disease may be at the root of a complex web of medical and psychological issues, but the entire person needs attention and healing. In Harry's case, the root was inexorable, but there was still a lot the medical community could do to support the boy who was living with it.

PAUL

I would spend the next fifteen years completing my education and getting established as a physician, and each time I met a new patient with CF, I thought of Harry and hoped I'd be able to do justice to his memory with empathetic medical care. Near the end of those years, I met the patient who made me realize hypnosis might be a critical component in whole-child healing.

From my earliest days in medicine, I had almost daily opportunities to see how anxiety and fear could exacerbate symptoms, but it was a patient named Paul who opened my eyes to the possibility that an entire field of care for these children—perhaps for most children— was being ignored. Even now, decades after our first encounter and years since his perilous health gave out, I still think of him nearly every day.

"Paul is the most allergic patient I've ever encountered," his pediatrician warned when he asked me to consult on the case of a patient hospitalized with severe breathing complications. "He's nearly died twice after exposure to milk products."

Months later in my office, the tall, thin, pale seventeen-year-old told me he'd suffered a severe asthma attack after smelling a cheeseburger. I'd never heard of the airborne aroma of a food (in this case, one of the milk products Paul avoided at all costs) causing a grave reaction, and my first thought was to tell him to go see his allergist. But even at that early point in my career, I had learned to take my patients at their word and proceed from there.

With that in mind, I suggested we try an experiment.

"Imagine there's a grill, over there," I pointed into the hall. "There are burgers on it, cheese melting on top. I'd like you to imagine eating one. Can you do that?" I knew this was something Paul could never do in real life because of his allergies. As he concentrated, he swallowed slowly. Within a few seconds he began breathing faster. His nostrils flared. His eyes widened, and he appeared to be struggling to inhale, which stopped me in my tracks.

I'd helped create the cheeseburger in his imagination, but the boy in front of me appeared to be suffering from an extreme reaction, one that, if allowed to worsen, could have catastrophic consequences.

"STOP IT!" I exclaimed.

Mercifully, he did. I thought he might have been joking, but Paul looked as frightened as I felt, and he insisted his symptoms had been real—just as real as the ones that had landed him in the hospital many times in his young life.

A LAYER OF GLASS

Paul and I sat together, both wrestling with what had happened. One thing I knew for sure: he hadn't feigned the attack. Was Paul's imagination uniquely powerful? Or was there some kind of power in my suggestion (which seemed unlikely since all I'd done was ask him to think of a cheeseburger)? Had he thought his way into what appeared to be a near medical emergency? I considered the possibility, dismissed it, and then circled back. What other explanation made sense?

"Are you OK?" I asked.

Paul nodded. "I'm fine now. But I don't get it."

The sum total of my knowledge of hypnosis at that moment was based on what a physician friend had told me. She'd done workshop training but hadn't even used it with her patients yet. Still, I knew hypnosis can be triggered with imagery. That idea fit, albeit oddly, with what had just occurred.

On a hunch, I decided to test the possibility that imagery was at work by suggesting that Paul experiment with a different kind of image.

"I'd like to try something, if it's OK?" I asked.

He nodded.

"Good," I began, "put your hand out, palm up."

He extended his right hand.

"Now, close your eyes and imagine there's a glass plate covering it," I said. "The glass is pretty thick."

"OK," he said, following the instruction.

"Now, tell me if you feel me touching your hand," I said. I brushed his palm with my finger, and he made no response.

"Anything?" I asked.

He shook his head.

I pinched his hand lightly. "Do you feel that?"

"No," he replied softly.

I reached into a pocket for my Swiss army knife and folded out its sharp-tipped corkscrew. I applied the tip rather forcefully to his hand.

"How about now? Can you feel this?"

"No," he replied even more softly. He was completely calm, breathing easily, showing no sign of the respiratory crisis that had ended just minutes earlier.

I was vaguely familiar with the phenomenon of kids who can use this kind of hypnotic technique to help themselves overcome needle phobia, but I had never seen it in person. Still skeptical, I asked Paul to extend his left hand and open his palm. "Can you feel this?" I asked as I pressed the corkscrew into his left palm—the one not covered by an imaginary plate.

"Ouch!" he protested, snapping his arm back.

Huh. I asked Paul to open his eyes, and he gave me a glare.

"You really didn't feel it when I touched your right hand?" I asked.

"No," he replied. "No, but you hurt my left hand!"

"I'm sorry. Are you OK?"

"It's no big deal," he said. "Just thought you'd want to know that hurt. On the left."

There was no question in that moment, or in the year that followed during my relationship with Paul, that his immune system was abnormal and his allergic response alarmingly intense. But after that day I couldn't let go of my wonder about what had happened or the essential question it raised: "If you can think your way into disease, can you think your way out?"

THE NEXT NATURAL STEP

Seeing how amenable Paul was to suggestion, I offered to refer him to a psychologist in my community who could teach him to use hypnosis. I hoped that instruction might help him learn how to control some of his scary breathing problems. At the time I didn't realize that Paul's anxiety was a major cause of his medical issues or that hypnosis could provide him with tools to better cope with it.

Paul made it clear he was interested in the hypnosis but not the referral.

"I don't want another doctor," he told me. "I've got plenty of those. Besides, I trust you."

I had no idea whether it was possible for me to facilitate hypnosis, but I promised to look into it. I'd majored in psychology in college and was interested, but that certainly didn't qualify me as a practitioner. I didn't want to waste Paul's time or complicate his already troubling issues.

I reached out to Dr. David Keith, a friend and child psychiatrist at my medical center, to ask what he thought of the idea. Dr. Keith was a well-respected clinician who was unconventional in his therapeutic approach, focusing on whole-family dynamics rather than individual work with the children in his care. I trusted both his expertise and his instincts.

Because we had done a number of family therapy sessions together for families who had children with CF, Dr. Keith had frequently observed my interactions with patients and parents. Afterward, he'd encouraged me to start providing therapeutic counseling within the framework of conventional medical treatment, which I had done.

When I asked about Paul, he expressed confidence that my experience as a clinician working with critically ill patients would guide me in assessing whether this therapy had value (or not) for my patient. Dr. Keith told me that he felt all good clinicians use psychotherapy as part of their practice, whether they realize they're doing it or not. He also promised that if hypnosis raised psychological issues that were out of my depth, he'd see Paul himself.

Lastly, he suggested that learning more about hypnosis would likely make me a better physician for *all* my patients and that it would enhance my communication skills.

With the knowledge that I had well-qualified backup, I told Paul we could work together to find out whether he could help himself. I cautioned him that I was not an expert in hypnosis or psychiatry, saying, "There's a lot that I don't know about this."

"That's what I like about working with you," he said with a slight grin. "I don't have to worry about you overanalyzing me."

His enthusiasm and Dr. Keith's reassurance were enough encouragement. I bought and borrowed several books on clinical hypnosis and dove in.

LEARNING TO RELAX

Paul and I met for the first of many hypnosis sessions with two hours on the clock and uncertain expectations.

Often, the first step of therapeutic hypnosis is relaxation, and there are many different ways to get there. Slow, deliberate breathing can help; so can focusing inward or on a fixed object or location. For Paul's first session, we agreed that he would think of the most relaxing place he could imagine and I would help him figure out how to get there with hypnosis. After having read a number of techniques, I settled on one that seemed like a simple and logical "recipe" for relaxation.

In my office, I asked Paul to close his eyes, to breathe deeply, and to imagine himself descending a staircase as I counted slowly down from ten. He nodded silently, and I watched intently for any response I could interpret as I slowly spoke the numbers. I noticed that his facial muscles relaxed when I got to seven, his shoulders slumped at six, and his eyelids flickered at four. When I got to zero, I suggested to Paul that he had reached the bottom of the staircase, where he imagined a door. Behind that door he could find a special place, one that made him feel relaxed and well. Once there, I invited him to describe what he perceived to me.

In the years since I began practicing hypnosis, I've had children tell me their relaxation places are as far away as Mars, Rivendell, or Hogwarts and as close as their own beds or backyards. Many choose the ocean or the mountains. The beach was a particular favorite among my patients in chilly upstate New York. Paul found his hypnosis home on the water. From the first day we practiced, he imagined being immersed in the same scene when he reached the bottom of the stairs. He was alone in a small boat, fishing at the center of a deep, clear lake. When I asked what he could see, he described the glint of the sun reflecting off the blue water. When I asked how it smelled, he said the air was clean and he could smell the pine needles on the trees along the shoreline. I wondered whether there was anything he could taste, and he smiled and said he had a crisp green apple. Asked what he felt, Paul described a warm breeze, and then, with a slight wave of his hand, he reported that the water was cool—too cold for swimming. He said he could drop a pebble in it and watch the ripples spread across the water toward land.

It certainly sounded like Paul's mind had conjured a truly relaxing, idyllic place to experience hypnosis. Some kids decide to change their location as they progress in hypnosis, to move on to spaces that better suit their wants, but Paul's lake quickly became his refuge—a peaceful place where he felt in control of every aspect of his experience.

During that first session, after Paul described what he experienced with all five senses, I talked him through imagining his body relaxing from head to toe.

My goal for this first session was to help Paul feel more capable of managing his own anxiety—to give him a tool he could use at will to relax. If it worked, I hoped we could move on to controlling his perception of pain in future sessions.

I told Paul he could stay in hypnosis for as long as he liked and to let me know when he was ready to come back by nodding his head. After five minutes, he nodded slowly.

"Great," I said. "Let me count you back up the staircase from your lake. By the time you reach the top, you can come completely back here." As I counted, Paul ascended the stairs slowly and then opened his eyes without being told to do so.

"What was that like?" I asked.

"It seemed so real," he exclaimed. "It felt like I was there for hours."

"Do you feel relaxed?"

He grinned. "I don't think I've ever been so relaxed in my life."

That's when I knew something important had just occurred.

Now alert, Paul looked calm and self-possessed—a far cry from the stressed-out young man he'd been in my office during the cheeseburger incident. I praised him for how quickly he'd figured out how to embrace the technique.

I shouldn't have been surprised by Paul's quick success. He'd been dealing with the medical and psychological complications of his condition for all of his short life, and he had the gift of a powerful imagination. Offered a potentially effective, relevant tool—a painless one that made him feel more in control of his experience and his symptoms—it should have been obvious that he would grab it.

Paul was eager to practice going through the steps of hypnosis at home, and within a few days he reported that he could self-hypnotize, transporting himself to his calm place any time he wanted or needed to. In the months to come, he honed this ability to the point that he could go to the lake in his mind for just a few minutes and come back as calm and relaxed as if he'd been gone for hours.

One of the most striking things about the early days of this process was the ease with which Paul learned to practice hypnosis and how intuitive it felt for me to guide it—as if it were a natural extension of the work I'd been doing as a doctor for more than a decade. I'd had passing experiences with a number of other mind-body healing techniques, including biofeedback, acupuncture, and yoga. Even though each has remarkable benefits, if Paul had chosen any of those disciplines, it likely would have taken him weeks or months to make significant headway.

Helping Paul achieve the kind of peace he found in the center of his lake felt like worthwhile work, and over the following months we continued to practice and learn from each other once or twice a week. I could not have known during the first hypnosis sessions that those hours would eventually lead to an evolution of my understanding of medicine or that my patient Paul, like my friend Harry before him, would become a catalyst of change not only in my life but also in the lives of thousands of patients I would see in the future.

WHAT YOU CAN DO ON YOUR OWN

Even without guided hypnosis, children can learn to recenter themselves by thinking of a calm place where they feel safe and comfortable. To foster this ability, talk with your child about the place where they feel relaxed. Ask them what they would experience in that place with each of their senses. What might they see, hear, smell, feel, and taste? Encourage your child to describe the place with as many details as possible. When they finish their description, ask them what they notice feels different. Are they more relaxed? Has any discomfort improved? Remind your child that whenever they want to feel better, they can return to their relaxing place.

2

The Mystery and History
Hypnosis All around Us

The concept of hypnosis is nearly as old as the history of civilization, part of global spiritual and healing traditions dating back to ancient Egypt, Persia, China, India, and Rome. From relaxation methods to sleep rituals, from psychological "cleansing" of sickness to use as an effective anesthetic (well before the advent of ether), hypnotic techniques have long been the tools of healers around the world. They are part of the history of hypnosis but also part of the problem with our understanding of it. Peppered among the ancient (and even the not-so-ancient) stories of hypnosis are references to the occult, to mind control, to witchcraft—all decidedly bad PR that does nothing to foster confidence in it as a modern-day medical tool.[1]

In Greek mythology, for example, Hypnos was the god of sleep, the child of night and darkness. The therapy with Hypnos's namesake can be a source of healing and light, but we tend to fixate—like his origin story does—on the dark side.

Why? First, because it's part of human nature to eye things we don't understand with suspicion—especially those we cannot quickly confirm with our own senses. The art of hypnosis is complex, and the science is something we are just beginning to understand after a couple thousand years of guessing (sometimes quite wildly) at how and why it works.

Equally influential in our perception of hypnosis are the unsubtle cues we routinely encounter about it, especially as children. Remember *The Jungle Book?* In both movie versions (though not in the original Rudyard Kipling story), the massive python Kaa uses a soothing, meditative voice, arresting eyes, and the slow-rolling repetition of the words "Trust in me" to hypnotize the child Mowgli. As the snake unhinges its jaw to swallow him whole, Mowgli is rescued—but the scene, with its insinuation that hypnosis is a power used for evil, leaves a lasting impression. That is but one negative reference. The Pied Piper of Hamlin and the witches in the movie *Hocus Pocus* use forms of hypnosis to lure children from their families. Evil Jafar uses it to manipulate the sultan in *Aladdin*. Wormtongue relies on hypnotic technique to keep King Theoden under his thumb in *The Lord of the Rings*. Even the *Captain Underpants* crowd has gotten in on the act, invoking a magic hypnotizing ring to gain control over a character's mind.

The sordid depictions carry over into popular entertainment for adults, from the sinister hypnotist in *Svengali* to the hypnotized assassin at the center of *The Manchurian Candidate* to a slew of B-level horror films that distort hypnosis to seem like the ideal tool to corrupt moral people for evil.

All these portrayals share the common characterization of the hypnotized individual as a victim, and it's worth noting that of all the misconceptions about hypnosis, this is the one that riles my patients and their parents the most. It is the opposite of the truth of their experience, and as you'll see in the details of their cases, hypnosis therapy has helped them claim more personal power—over their bodies, their feelings, and their relationships—than previously seemed possible.

ANYBODY'S CLAIM

Disappointingly, the image problem saddling hypnosis doesn't end at the movies. One of the biggest obstacles clinical hypnosis practitioners face is the fact that anyone can hang out a shingle or print up a business card claiming to be a hypnotist. It's not like putting an MD or PhD or

RN after your name—credentials that reflect years of study, practice, and oversight. The terms *hypnotist* and even *hypnotherapist* are largely unregulated. That makes it all too easy for anyone new to this idea to lump a highly trained physician who studies hypnotic technique for its therapeutic value together with, for example, a stage performer who convinces audience volunteers to bark like dogs or fall asleep on command. It is the latter sketchy practitioners and performers who lead many in the public to believe hypnosis therapy amounts to quackery.

Of all the concerns about whether therapeutic hypnosis is right for your family, finding a qualified practitioner is the easiest to address. The rule of thumb patients and parents should follow is simple: any person who is qualified to treat a particular condition with hypnosis should be equally qualified to treat the same condition without it. If your child has a medical or psychiatric diagnosis (or an as-yet-undiagnosed medical or psychological condition), a medical or mental health professional is the right person to handle that case. Seek out one of these professionals who is also trained in hypnosis therapy. It takes an average of eleven to fourteen years of formal education to become a doctor but only several weeks of training for someone with a medical or mental health background to become competent at hypnosis (though, just as for other types of medical care, practitioners utilizing hypnosis improve their abilities the more they study and practice). Feel free to ask about your practitioner's experience but feel confident that his or her medical training is sufficient insurance that this therapy will be offered in a safe, constructive manner. It is my fervent hope that with each passing year more medical professionals will make this training a priority so they can better meet their patients' psychological needs.

REALITY CHECK

Because of the sometimes mysterious and negative associations hypnosis carries, discussion about its role in healing sometimes starts with establishing what it is *not*. Generally speaking, hypnosis is none of the things it's depicted to be in entertainment. It is not a tool for mind control. It is not sleep. It is not controlled by others. All effective therapeutic hypnosis, even if it is guided, is self-hypnosis. Without the participation of the person who enters this state, it doesn't work and, more important for our purposes, it has no therapeutic value. As a clinician, it's part of my role to help children learn to be confident in their control of the hypnotic process. I can tell you with the certainty of a physician who routinely works with teenagers (who can be uniquely and dedicatedly resistant to ideas that are not their own) that without their active participation in the process, therapeutic hypnosis doesn't happen.

WHAT HYPNOSIS *IS*

At its essence, hypnosis is a distinct plane of inward attention, a more intense and narrow focus than our conscious level of awareness in our daily lives. It's a state in which distractions fall away, in which the individual is capable of being absorbed in a thought or a task or an effort to problem-solve. It is a state the hypnotized person achieves, not something that's forced on him or her.

In truth, we can find the seeds of hypnosis scattered throughout our everyday lives, even when we're not looking for them. You can recognize hints of hypnotic suggestion when a teacher uses positive language to lead a class in a creative exercise; when a parent lulls a child to sleep with a familiar bedtime story or kisses a boo-boo to make it better; when a doctor makes a suggestion that sticks with a patient, influencing his or her perception. Many of us (and especially many of our children) frequently take ourselves into the realm of hypnosis as well. Anytime you daydream, or let your mind wander while you do rote work, or drift into a memory when you hear a particular song or smell a unique aroma, you are in the vicinity of that hypnotic state. In it, you are more amenable to suggestions, because the conscious mind is engaged in a focused activity that distracts it from skeptical thoughts.

Many of the therapeutic objectives achievable with the help of reaching this state involve a common accomplishment: greater self-regulation on the part of the child. This can come in the form of being able to breathe deeply and calmly in times of physical or emotional distress; it can be managing the perception of pain; it can be visualizing outcomes in which the child attains a goal. It can also be the ability to overcome functional symptoms (medical symptoms with no known physical causes), things like habit cough, anxiety-related stomachaches and headaches, and enuresis (bedwetting). It can even be helpful in patients with physical disease whose symptoms worsen because of psychological distress—like shortness of breath that develops because of anxiety in a patient with asthma. Each of these outcomes is a victory for the child, as well as a step toward independence. Because therapeutic hypnosis puts many patients on paths to thinking and acting on their own, it can work small miracles for their self-esteem.

These outcomes aren't just part of my extensive experience. Many of them are well documented. Clinical studies have shown therapy with hypnosis to help inhibit nausea in children undergoing chemotherapy. They've shown it to be superior to medication in treating childhood migraines. They've proven it effective in curbing habit problems like hair pulling. They've demonstrated its usefulness in treating asthma, irritable bowel syndrome, and Tourette syndrome. Numerous studies track its effectiveness in managing pain, anxiety, and multiple sleep disorders.[2]

It is important to note that entering a hypnotic state is not a medical treatment. Rather, therapy involves directing a patient toward a therapeutic goal while in hypnosis. As a shorthand in this book, I use the term *hypnosis* as applied clinically to mean achievement of a hypnotic state *and* use of therapeutic suggestions.

What hypnosis *is*, in terms of what happens in the brain and nervous system during the process, is a different kind of question—one that modern neuroscientists are just beginning to understand. Today they can demonstrate that hypnosis is a mental state distinct from being awake or asleep. Using the technologies of functional magnetic resonance imaging and electroencephalography, multiple studies have shown changes in neural activity during hypnosis, with some activity centers and pathways "lighting up" and others slowing down. Through this we can see evidence of increases in focused attention and emotional control as well as less activity in areas of the brain that we associate with self-consciousness.[3]

All of this ties in directly with the evidence I see every day that by learning to use hypnosis and applying themselves to particular problems, children can overcome and eliminate habitual actions that they might otherwise believe are beyond their control.

COMMON QUESTIONS

A number of issues inevitably arise in any consideration of clinical hypnosis, and I'd like to address a couple of the big ones before delving into individual cases:

- Hypnosis or meditation: Hypnosis differs from other mind-body approaches to wellness, but because it is outwardly similar to meditation, the two processes are often confused. While both hypnosis and meditation involve changing one's mind-set from usual conscious awareness, meditation involves a singular focus (such as the breath or a mantra) in order to increase awareness of the moment. In contrast, hypnosis involves imagery and suggestions made by a clinician (or self-suggestions), and its purpose is to prompt change involving specific goals. Each of these methods is useful in its own right, and they may complement one another when both are used.

- Hypnotizability: Studies have demonstrated that the majority of kids are highly hypnotizable, while adults are less so.[4] In my own experience, I've found that almost anyone who *wants* to be hypnotized is capable of it. The converse is equally true: people who do not want to be hypnotized generally won't be. Several times I've met patients who are resistant to the idea of hypnosis—and it doesn't work for them. When their circumstances change—perhaps because some other treatment fails or simply because their symptoms persist—and they then ask for hypnosis, it works.

- Magic or medicine: Some stage hypnosis is just that—staged—but not all of it. For centuries, performers have been implementing hypnosis for its entertainment value. Early practitioners described it in terms of "animal magnetism" and "thought projection," but there's no evidence either of those things is true. Scottish surgeon James Braid, one of the best-documented early pioneers of using hypnosis in medicine, insisted a different concept was at work—one that presumed a combination of mental focus and suggestion. He used the term *monoideism*, meaning intense focus on one idea—a name that's an apt description for what we still call hypnosis to this day.[5]

  Often, when real hypnosis is happening on a stage, the process starts before the show with deliberate screening of audience members. Hypnotists look for individuals who are engaged, interested, and imaginative—all indicators of a willingness and ability to use hypnosis. Regardless of how they're selected, audience participants are volunteers, so when a stage hypnotist tells them to fall asleep at a finger snap or hand clap, the control that's implied there is something they have embraced rather than had pushed on them.

  Among medical practitioners who use hypnosis as a therapeutic tool, the logical question is "Is it a good idea for experts in hypnotic technique to use it for entertainment purposes?"

  Often the answer is no: first, because hypnosis can be a uniquely powerful therapy that should only be used with the well-being of the hypnotized individual at heart; second, because using this skill to entertain an audience rather than to empower an individual may give volunteers the impression they can be controlled or are weak willed. This is not true. The ability to become hypnotized is a skill, not a weakness.

- Physical versus mental symptoms: Among the first and most vigorous objections to hypnosis is the idea that its success implies illness might be all in a patient's mind. Nothing could be further than the truth. This is a deeply complex issue—one we'll explore in depth in later chapters, but it bears addressing up front. Can you think your way to

shrinking a tumor? Can you think away a life-threatening allergy? A
genetic lung defect? The answer is obviously no. There's no thinking
your way out of some conditions. But illness is far bigger than the
genetic, chemical, or other physical factors that contribute to chronic
health conditions. The ways these manifest are complicated, with
symptoms over which the brain does have some control intimately
tangled up with those over which it does not. In my experience, there
are almost always ways to help sick children feel better and stronger,
even when there is no cure for their condition. In my practice, I've
been able to teach kids how to use hypnosis to give them a measure
of control over the many aspects of their physical and psychological troubles that *can* be managed. Over that time, I've seen hypnosis
help children as young as three and as old as twenty who struggle
to breathe, children who can't sleep, children with eating disorders,
pain, migraines, seizures, anxiety, and chronic disease. It has helped
kids who can't concentrate in class and those who live with paralyz-
ing phobias. Hypnosis has even been of value—maybe of particular
value—to those who are severely or even terminally ill.

The benefits of hypnosis-facilitated therapy for these patients
have extended beyond the physical and into the psychological and
spiritual, building confidence, positivity, and resilience. They've included the empowerment of children with all kinds of health issues to
feel more in control of their own minds, bodies, and circumstances.
They've sometimes led to the reduction or elimination of medications. They've kept kids out of operating rooms, put them back in
classrooms, and given them the tools they need to face their problems
and feel competent to do so.

I never thought, when I decided to devote fourteen years of my life
to studying first general medicine, then pediatrics, and then pulmonology, that one day I'd be building and sharing a body of clinical experience showing hypnosis to be the most powerful, underutilized tool in
pediatric care today. And yet that's where I find myself now—beating

a drum for an invaluable and overlooked treatment. Children deserve the opportunity to receive gentle, thoughtful, empowering, and effective treatment in whatever form it's available. Beyond any doubt, hypnosis therapy offers all of those things.

WHAT YOU CAN DO ON YOUR OWN

Become aware of hypnosis in everyday life: Think about the subtle (and not-so-subtle) ways hypnosis regularly interfaces with your daily life. Think of how you rely on routines or habits to easily complete various tasks throughout the day. This is an example of allowing your conscious mind to focus on something other than the routine tasks, which is a hypnotic phenomenon. Consider all the things your mind processes while you are walking or driving (when you are not actively engaging in those activities).

As a parent, think about the ways you explain things to children that engage their conscious imaginations and tap into their impressionable subconscious sides. If you pray or meditate or do yoga or work out, think about how those activities affect your breathing and heart rate, how they alter your focus and the way you feel. Consider how each of these things brings you or your child closer to a state of focused, inward attention. In doing so, recognize that hypnosis isn't a wild, crazy, or foreign experience—it's an aspect of everyday living that might just be the missing piece to the health plan you and your child's doctor have devised that's coming up short.

Teddy Goes to Mars

The Interwoven Nature of Physical and Psychological Symptoms

One of the first questions that arises when you consider the potential healing power of hypnosis is where we draw the line between symptoms rooted in physical causes and those that are psychological. This is something I answer based on years of treating children with chronic and debilitating diseases: there is no hard line. Physical health and mental health are deeply interwoven. The vast majority of people with chronic illness, for example, develop psychological issues that can affect the severity of their symptoms. This is part of the normal experience of sickness, and it leads to changes in the way patients' symptoms present. There is even some evidence that chronic pain can lead to changes in the actual structure of the brain and how the brain responds to future stressful situations.[1] Further, patients with functional disorders—symptoms lacking an identifiable organic origin—suffer just as much as those whose symptoms have a clear physiologic cause. Any doctor or other health care provider must consider how psychology might impact each patient; otherwise we are not fully doing our jobs.

When I became aware of therapeutic hypnosis, my patients included kids who were medically fragile because of identifiable physical causes—among them muscular atrophy, anatomical abnormalities, and atypical reactions to allergens—but those same patients were also impacted every day by anxiety and stress, anger and fear. In order to be a good physician, I owed it to them to consider and help alleviate all the potential roots of their distress.

After helping Paul practice hypnosis for nearly a year and becoming a more finessed guide, I began offering this therapy to patients with a variety of symptoms. What followed, beginning with a boy named Teddy, was the revelation that hypnosis could help children avoid invasive and expensive procedures. Suddenly I wasn't thinking of it simply in terms of something extra I could give my patients; I was realizing it was a game changer in terms of both diagnosis and treatment.

QUESTIONING THE PROTOCOL

Teddy was eleven when he bounded into my office in a Ninja Turtles T-shirt. He was stocky and freckled, with wavy dark hair and a quick, shy smile. I noted that in the office he moved and spoke with energy and openness, but I knew from the medical history I'd received that for months he'd been shuffling back and forth from his sixth-grade classroom to the school nurse's office because he couldn't breathe. Each time it happened, he'd begin to feel a lump in his throat and then sense it blocking his breath. His face would redden as he sucked in air, trying to force it around the blockage.

Teddy described the incidents to me, sounding fearful and frustrated at how powerless he felt each time the lump in his throat returned. The problem always resolved with rest, but he was anxious and embarrassed. His parents worried about the day-to-day impacts of their son's episodes, and they worried even more about their root cause. Did he have a tumor? Was he suffering from a disease that might get worse? Would he have to live with this alarming problem for the rest of his life?

I tested Teddy's breathing on a pulmonary-function machine, asking him to blow as long and hard as he could. There, in the quiet safety of my office, his breathing pattern was normal. Based on my medical training, the next step in diagnosing the problem would have been a barium-swallow X-ray of his neck and chest. The test would allow me to see if any abnormality might be causing the symptoms. Teddy would swallow a liquid dye, and the X-ray would indicate any pressure points on his esophagus (food pipe). It was possible he had irregular blood vessels that were compressing his airway and food pipe or that something, like a bone, was lodged there. Those things are rare, but rare happens.

If the X-ray was clear, protocol would dictate sending Teddy for a pH probe study. He'd have a thin tube placed down his food pipe to his stomach. He would have to skip a day of school because he'd have the temporary tube sticking out of his nose. A positive probe test would indicate that acid reflux might be causing irritation of his throat and a sensation that it was blocked. In that case, he would be treated with antacid pills. A negative result would lead to scheduling a bronchoscopy—during which Teddy would be placed under anesthesia while a large tube was inserted into his throat to visually inspect his airways for abnormalities.

All of those procedures were part of a standard approach to treatment for Teddy's symptom, and for my first decade of medical practice, I would have followed them in order, looking for a "smoking gun"— physical evidence of a root problem. Despite that experience, I didn't order any tests for Teddy at our first appointment. Even though he was uncomfortable, he was in no immediate danger. The timing of his episodes—only during school hours—made me suspect there was a psychologically based component to them. If there were something wrong with him physically, it should have caused him to develop symptoms at different times and locations. With that in mind, I proposed to him and to his parents that before we went down the expensive and invasive path of diagnostic tests, we might try something gentler and simpler. I could teach Teddy hypnosis, and together we could work on finding a way to resolve his symptoms. If they were functional—rooted in some unidentified psychological component—we could likely achieve a cure. If they were not and hypnosis didn't help, then we'd continue with medical investigations. Either way, we had nothing to lose but a little time.

Teddy and his parents were open to the idea and wanted to know when we could start.

In our first session, Teddy arrived eager but also obviously nervous. I told him we needed to talk a little about what hypnosis is and is not before we got started. I was learning with each patient who was offered hypnosis what their misperceptions of it were and how I could set their minds at ease.

"First of all," I explained, "hypnosis doesn't involve one person controlling another person's mind. I won't control you, and you won't be able to control your friends."

He exhaled audibly, nodded, and expressed a bit of disappointment that he would not be able to make his friends do things.

"I'm never going to tell you what you have to do," I continued. "And even if I did, you would always be able to refuse. Second, hypnosis is not sleep. When you're doing it, you'll be awake, you'll know what's going on, and you'll be able to stop at any time. You will be in control of your experience."

Teddy nodded in understanding.

"Finally, hypnosis is not unusual. You see a lot of crazy things on TV and in movies about it, but most of those are made up. Most people do hypnosis in some form almost every day. For example, do you ever daydream and picture yourself taking part in something you're going to do after school?"

"Yeah?"

"Using your imagination that way is a kind of hypnosis," I said.

He looked at me with wide eyes.

"Can you imagine what your favorite song might sound like?" I asked.

He nodded. "Yes. Can't everyone?"

"No, some people can't hear a melody unless it's playing. But you can, and that's another example of you doing hypnosis without realizing it. This is really something you already know how to do very well," I summed up. "I'm going to teach you how to use that state of mind to achieve some things you didn't know you could do."

When patients tell me they can imagine things easily, they usually turn out to be gifted with hypnosis. Teddy was no exception.

He had heard enough. Sitting on the edge of his chair, he said, "Let's do it."

FRIED EGGS AND COLD RIVERS

Teddy told me he liked to imagine himself going to outer space, so I suggested he take a spaceship to Mars in his first session. I encourage my patients who practice hypnosis to imagine what they might perceive with all of their senses in a relaxing place of their choice. It helps make the experience feel as real as possible and enhances relaxation. This is how most of my patients achieve a hypnotic state, and for many of them the resultant relaxation is sufficient to improve their symptoms. For others, once they are in hypnosis, I offer additional suggestions that can help.

Teddy reported that he saw red mountains. He heard the air in his spacesuit. When I asked whether he could taste anything, he said he tasted chocolate milk, which he could drink through a straw concealed in a compartment in the suit. At the edge of the room, Teddy's mom smiled at this comment but didn't say anything. Confident Teddy was quite good at this part of the process, I then walked him through relaxing from head to toe while on this imaginary Mars.

After I counted him back out of hypnosis, Teddy reported that the experience had seemed real, that Mars was just the way he'd thought it would be. I had to chuckle at this assessment—it seemed he'd momentarily forgotten the Mars in his session and the one in his imagination were one and the same.

"I want to do it again," he said eagerly and closed his eyes.

I waited, and when he opened his eyes a moment later, I asked where he had gone.

"To the moon."

I complimented Teddy on his ability to imagine and then asked if he could imagine himself having trouble breathing as he did sometimes at school. He said he'd try; a moment later, he said he felt the lump in his throat.

I could see that his breathing was changing but knew he was in no danger. Rather than comment on the strain I was hearing as he inhaled, I asked him what the lump looked like.

"Like an egg," he said. "A big one."

I asked him how he might get rid of the egg.

"Um, I guess I could eat it," he said. "I could fry it and eat it."

I suggested that he should go ahead and do it. Somewhere in the recesses of his mind, Teddy went about this task, imagining the steps in order. His body visibly relaxed.

A moment later, when I asked about his breathing, he said it was fine.

I told Teddy he could use hypnosis as a tool any time he wanted, but in order to get good at it, he'd need to practice. He promised to relax and focus and go to Mars every day until the next time I saw him.

"And you can fry and eat that egg any time you need," I added.

"I get it," he said, and I suspected he did.

When I next saw Teddy, a week later, he reported that he'd practiced every day and been to other planets besides Mars. Clearly, his vivid imagination made self-hypnosis feel like a game to him, and he was very good at it.

Prior to our first meeting, Teddy had experienced an obstruction in his throat and breathing difficulties almost every day at school. When I asked about the intervening week, he reported it had happened just once (his mom, incredulous, reported the same).

We talked about the one "lump" that had occurred and how imagining eating it hadn't been enough to clear it away. I said it must have been a big one, and Teddy nodded, saying it was more like a boulder than an egg.

"If you ever experience that again, how can you clear it?" I asked.

Teddy thought about this for a minute and then informed me that boulders get washed away by rivers. We agreed that he could swallow and imagine the mighty flow of a river clearing the stones out of his way.

That was the end of that complaint. Teddy continued to practice hyp-nosis on a regular basis, and in the weeks that followed, he didn't suffer any breathing difficulties at school. During our three-month follow-up, he informed me that he no longer had a breathing problem, so he was also going to stop practicing hypnosis. At nine months, I spoke with Teddy and his mom together, and we all agreed he was ready to be dis-charged from my care.

Teddy's outcome—achieved without medication or invasive medical tests—was shockingly simple once he learned to trust his own power to control his symptoms. This was possible only because doctor, parents, and child understood that physical and mental perception are inti-mately intertwined. It is my firm belief that parents need to recognize that the psychological manifestations associated with any serious or long-term illness are equally as important as the physical ones. They can cause just as much or even more suffering.

The path we took to get to Teddy's outcome gave me a lot to think about as well. A year earlier, I would have subjected this child to a battery of uncomfortable and expensive tests, which would not have revealed a physical problem. Ultimately, I'm confident I would have reached the same conclusion if I'd taken that route: that Teddy's breath-ing obstruction was a functional symptom. The question is: How long would it have taken me to get there? And what would that process have cost my patient and his family—in time, in dollars, and in physical dis-comfort? In addition, before I learned about hypnosis, I was able to offer little treatment for a functional symptom other than reassurance that it did not require medical therapy. Such reassurance sometimes helped patients to feel better, but for some patients this was insufficient, and they ended up with ongoing discomfort that sometimes prompted them to go from physician to physician in an effort to find a medical solution that was not there.

As time went on, I would come to realize that Teddy's case was not as exceptional as it felt in the moment. In fact, before long I would be routinely and safely diagnosing and treating many children without the need for invasive and expensive procedures. Not every case could be resolved with hypnosis, but being open to it as a diagnostic tool was the beginning of a sea change in my understanding of the practice of pulmonary medicine.

SIGNS OF EMOTIONS AT WORK

Teddy's case was in part defined by the catch-22 of his physical symptoms and emotional response (and vice versa). Beyond doubt, his fear and anxiety played a role in his breathing difficulties. Many children's symptoms can be caused or aggravated by emotions, but parents struggle to understand what role emotions play.

We know that emotions can not just skew perception of symptoms but even cause them to appear. How many of us have experienced a headache, stomachache, or chest pain during a stressful time? How many of us have shed tears of joy? There's a reason the word *feelings* applies to both bodily and emotional experience.

Less often recognized is the fact that emotions can alter even symptoms of medical illnesses such as asthma, diabetes, and hypertension. Stress can trigger an asthma attack, high blood sugar, and increased blood pressure. Conversely, calming can help your child's breathing improve and bring down blood sugar and blood pressure. This is why use of self-calming techniques such as hypnosis, slow deep breathing, and changing the way we think about life stressors can lead to improved health. The following clues, among others, suggest your child's emotions may be related to their physical symptom(s):

- Anxious appearance: If your child appears edgy or uncomfortable or displays other emotional reactions before or after they develop symptoms, then it is possible that their emotions are causing the problem. Regardless of the root cause, it's likely that these emotions are making the symptoms worse.
- Dizziness: This can be the result of breathing too fast because the child is upset or scared. Such emotions can worsen other symptoms.

- Globus reaction: Feeling something is stuck in the throat—sometimes called globus—is often the result of feeling anxious or overwhelmed.
- Palpitations: A complaint that the child can feel their heartbeat is often a mark of anxiety.
- Shakiness: This sometimes occurs as a result of release of adrenaline during stressful times.
- Tingling or numbness: These changes in sensory perception can occur in the arms or legs, typically happening in children who have been breathing too fast as a result of anxiety.
- Timely absence of symptoms: If symptoms disappear during sleep or when your child is distracted, psychological stress may be playing a role in their expression at other times.

WHAT YOU CAN DO ON YOUR OWN

While it's important to validate your child's symptoms or distress regardless of the origin of the problem, it's also valuable to encourage kids to consider their own power and resources to deal with things that are bothering them. Gently encourage your child to come up with ideas for resolution. Even if these ideas are simply hypothetical, they serve two immediate purposes. First, they open a discussion that allows your child to describe the problem in their own language, how they feel about it, and how they envision a possible solution. Your child may need some encouragement in coming up with creative solutions. Remember that the solutions do not have to be realistic. You might cue your child regarding how to think outside the box and employ their vivid imagination. Second, such a discussion creates an environment in which the child sees the possibility of an answer coming from within. The self-confidence boost this realization can effect is key to helping increase your child's resilience in the face of medical difficulties. Whenever possible, conduct these conversations with the attitude of an ally—someone who is respectful of the child's own power but stands ready to offer help and support.

Kayla's Cross-Country Trek

When Medical Therapy Isn't Working, There's a Reason

In Teddy's case, there was no downside to using hypnosis to first explore the possibility his symptoms were functional before reaching any
deeper into the medical toolbox. He wasn't in any immediate danger, all
medical options were on the table, and hypnosis could potentially save
him and his family a great deal of time and trouble.

Too often I meet patients whose cases have gone down a different
path, when doctors at a loss to resolve their symptoms try one invasive, expensive therapy after another without success. This was what
happened to Kayla, a middle school track athlete who came to see me
because she'd developed a perplexing crisis during almost every race.
She'd try to breathe in, and her vocal cords and voice box would constrict, limiting her air intake. Race after race she could barely finish
as she struggled to catch her breath. After a while, her episodes began
happening at other times—though they still almost always occurred at
moments when she was under extreme pressure to perform, such as
during big school tests.

This thirteen-year-old from Arkansas had been through a traumatic
and ineffective diagnostic and treatment gauntlet: multiple prescription medications and invasive testing, including a laryngoscopy and a
bronchoscopy, and even a tonsillectomy. Just before I met her, it was
suggested that Botox injections to the vocal cords might be helpful,

but her parents became leery of trying yet another uncomfortable and possibly dangerous therapy. They were desperate for effective help and deeply frustrated with the care she'd had thus far. Her father searched the internet for treatment of vocal cord problems and came across medical articles I had written about using hypnosis for breathing disorders.[1] Early in my hypnosis career, I didn't know anyone in Arkansas who could help this family, but I offered to see Kayla at the upstate New York medical center where I was practicing if her parents were willing to bring her.

Because Kayla's symptoms most often happened during high-stress race settings, I suspected the origin of her distressing and seemingly dangerous episodes had a psychological component. If the problem was the result of a physical issue alone, then it would likely occur at random times. The fact that she specifically struggled to inhale (as opposed to exhale) indicated vocal cord dysfunction (VCD) as the most likely diagnosis.

A COMMON BUT UNDERDIAGNOSED DISORDER

VCD was first identified as a separate diagnosis from asthma in the early 1980s, but its origins go back much further—at least as far as the insultingly named "hysterical croup" of the mid-1800s. VCD's symptoms are frequently confused with those of asthma because they both cause noisy breathing, but the VCD triggers are usually psychological, and the symptoms tend to be most prominent while patients are inhaling, whereas asthma tends to interfere with exhalation.[2]

Any serious respiratory symptom can have consequences, and because VCD incidents like the ones it seemed Kayla was experiencing involve the adduction (narrowing) of the vocal cords, they can create medical emergencies. I've treated patients with this diagnosis who've been rushed to the ER by ambulance and undergone extensive—largely ineffective—medical interventions to try to correct the problem. Failed treatments are often the first indication that what's happening to a child with this condition is different from the typical presentation of asthma.

In a typical asthma event, an inhaled rescue medication opens up airways and provides rapid relief. When the culprit is VCD, this is not a solution. Since many patients suffer from both asthma and VCD, these cases can present unique diagnostic challenges.

THE DIAGNOSTIC BLIND SIDE

Personally, I never diagnosed a single case of VCD until after I started doing hypnosis with Paul. How could I overlook it? The reason is not surprising: I didn't know it existed.

Whether you're a doctor, parent, or patient, if you are unaware of a condition, it's easy to overlook it—in fact, that's the most likely outcome. Consider an X-ray. Even a child with a rudimentary understanding of human anatomy can take a quick glance at a chest X-ray and recognize the big picture: spine, ribs, lungs, and the blurs of bodily organs. But how many of us can distinguish the aortic knob or the pulmonary trunk or the subtle shadows that might indicate abnormalities that require investigation? Most of us only see the things we know. In this case, that's the shape of a torso and the general outlines of bones and organs.

Similarly, when I first learned to listen for heart murmurs as a medical student, I never heard anything out of the ordinary. It takes time and attention, training, and an awareness of the different types of murmurs to be able to recognize the unique syncopation of a systolic or diastolic murmur. Without an understanding of what I was listening for, all I heard was, well, a heartbeat.

Early in my career, when I didn't know about VCD, I approached these mysterious cases through the lens of asthma triggers, always searching for a physical or an environmental factor as the root cause. I was looking for an additional problem in the body or an allergen, when I should have been considering the possibility of a psychological stressor.

Not long after I began recognizing and successfully treating VCD, another patient, Susan, was referred by a pediatrician who called to discuss the case. Her incidents had a pattern, he told me, adding that they almost always took place Wednesday through Friday. He, the family, the child, and her teachers had investigated every imaginable trigger at the school. The possibility was raised that perhaps the child was reacting in the middle of the week to a buildup of an allergic reaction to something in the school building. While this was possible, it seemed more likely that the trigger wasn't something in the building. In this case, it turned out to be something in the schedule—a class Susan believed was do-or-die for her to get into college that wasn't going well. The stress of the weekly Friday quiz became overwhelming as each week progressed. This girl was no more aware that these circumstances triggered her symptoms than the doctor who referred her, but somewhere along the way, she had experienced respiratory distress in that class. Through a series of adverse connections, her body learned an unconscious response that aggravated her vocal cords and caused her to struggle for air. Rather than looking for the obvious difference between this child's early- and late-week routines, both family and pediatrician sought a Sherlock Holmes–worthy trigger.

There are times when we encounter medical mysteries that are truly worthy of great detectives, but for this child, the culprit was a class she dreaded and feared and an unusual response that could be corrected without medications.

VCD is only one of countless diagnoses that contain critical psychological components. Doctors and other medical practitioners overlooking the psychological side of illness are essentially working impaired. We can all do a better job for our children if we presume their health issues are based in both the physical and the psychological realms.

A CORRECTIBLE CONDITION

Over the past decade, I've seen patients with VCD nearly every week. How do I know I'm right about their diagnoses? Because most of those patients are cured within a handful of hypnosis therapy sessions. Some, even kids who have suffered symptoms for months or years, are cured in a single appointment.

In many ways, Kayla's case was a textbook example of VCD: a high-achieving teenage girl struggling to inhale while experiencing the extreme stress of a competitive event. As she and her family became more alarmed and frightened by the incidents, Kayla's memories of previous occurrences became a factor in new ones, and they were no longer confined just to races.

Seeing this young family in my office—the petite girl sporting a ponytail and tracksuit, her parents holding hands as they kept watch over her—my own emotions were mixed. I felt regret for what they'd been through, for the unnecessary surgery Kayla had endured and the strain her condition had put on her family. I felt relief that they were going to get some answers. And as I explained to Kayla, I felt joy, because I was sure her condition could be resolved.

"I think your symptoms are the result of vocal cord dysfunction," I explained. "If I'm right, what's happening is that your voice box is closing as you try to breathe in. It's a condition that occurs sometimes when people are psychologically stressed. In your case, that's when you're pushing yourself to perform your best in competition. It is an unusual way your body has found to respond to that stress."

"You don't think I'm sick?" Kayla asked.

"I don't," I answered. "I think your vocal cords have adopted an unusual and bothersome response to extreme stress."

Kayla listened attentively as I continued. "The tightening of your vocal cords is your body's way of saying, 'I feel overwhelmed, and I need to slow down.'"

Kayla nodded and asked the question that mattered most: "Can it be fixed?"

"Yes," I replied. "As you've found out, asthma and allergy medications and even surgery didn't help. The way to fix this is to use the power of your imagination to help relax your vocal cords. I can teach you how to do it with hypnosis."

Both Kayla and her parents were open to the idea of hypnosis, especially since they'd come a long way and subjected her to much more difficult treatments in the past. Kayla was curious, asking why, if she could use her own imagination to control her symptom, she hadn't already done so. Why did she need hypnosis to achieve the result if it was within her power?

"That's a great question!" I said. "First of all, there are many things that are within our power that we don't realize. Did you know you could learn how to ride a bicycle before you were shown how? Also, remember how I told you that your body may feel overwhelmed by the competitions?"

Kayla sighed quietly and nodded. I continued, "Before the symptom can go away, we have to teach your body a better way to deal with the stress. Hypnosis can give your body a new way to respond."

Kayla listened carefully, and then she said she'd like to get started.

Within a few moments, she was describing her relaxing place—a clearing at the top of a mountain from which she could see miles out in every direction, smell and taste fresh berries, and feel a thick, woolly blanket wrapped around her shoulders. I guided her to relax her body, starting with her forehead and taking deep, deliberate breaths as she let tension go from her head to her toes. I asked her to notice how peaceful and in control she felt of her body and of her breathing.

"Congratulations," I said. "You have an excellent imagination. You have a powerful ability to achieve calm. This is a feeling you can achieve any time you want by returning to your relaxing place. All you have to do is practice getting there. When you do this every day for two weeks, your mind and body will start to remember how to do it without you having to work at it."

"Your mind is open to good suggestions right now," I continued, "and you can picture your vocal cords, how they are open and relaxed and how easy it is for you to fill your lungs with clean air."

Wanting to give her a memorable, physical association to augment her sense of control over her breathing, I suggested perhaps she could turn her wrist slightly to the right when she felt like her airway was narrowing and imagine that doing so would open the airway the same way adjusting the vents over a heating duct works. Before inviting Kayla to return from hypnosis, I told her that her enhanced suggestibility gave her an excellent opportunity to think positive thoughts and tell herself good things. She could tell herself she felt calm and strong and that she intended to carry that feeling throughout the day. She could tell herself she had learned to breathe deliberately, remaining in control of the whole process. She could tell herself to be confident in her abilities as an excellent runner and an excellent student.

Finally, I told Kayla I would count from one to five, and as I did so, she would feel more alert and aware of her surroundings with each ascending number. After I reached five, she would join me when she was ready so we could talk about what had happened and the next steps.

Kayla opened her eyes and smiled broadly.

"That was awesome," she said. "I totally get it."

And she did. As it turned out, this child who had been through months of futile and frustrating medical interventions was able to achieve resolution of her symptoms in a single session. By learning to feel confident in her control over her vocal cords, she became able to stop future breathing incidents before they caused any discomfort. Kayla went home committed to practicing the technique every day for a month, and in a follow-up email three months later, her mother informed me that not only was her daughter free of her breathing ailment, but she also was racing competitively on the track team again.

TOO SIMPLE A SOLUTION?

Cases like Kayla's, with quick and painless resolution, sometimes provoke skepticism about hypnosis. The fact is, this was a simple case because Kayla's problem was an interior issue. She put tremendous pressure on herself to perform, and she hated the resulting breathing problem. Part of what made her a classic patient with VCD was her high-performing attitude, and that same spirit made her an ideal patient to resolve her own issues. In my experience, more than almost anything, kids want to have some control over their circumstances. This is never more true than when they are at the mercy of medical symptoms they find scary, embarrassing, and inconvenient. Learning she was capable of controlling her own breathing problem was all Kayla needed to fully embrace the technique that put her in the driver's seat. Once she'd mastered it, she got on with her life.

Often, however, other factors are at work when kids exhibit functional symptoms. External problems require more investigation, more consideration, and more nuanced techniques to overcome. If the root of the problem is not something the child can directly control—perhaps a bullying problem or an illness in the family or a looming parental divorce—the solution isn't simply teaching the child to manage the symptom (though it's an excellent start).

AT A MINIMUM

Addressing patients' psychological needs concurrently with a medical workup helps spare many kids needless investigations that can be uncomfortable or even traumatic, costly, and time-consuming. Given the high prevalence of psychological influences in children with chronic symptoms, parents should demand that psychology be addressed as soon as major medical issues are excluded (which often can be determined by history and physical examination and without extensive testing). If your child is already undergoing medical therapy and not responding as expected, don't wait to seek out psychological interventions, including hypnosis. In addition, it's worth noting that medical therapy and hypnosis can complement one another. Even if your child responds well to treatment for a chronic issue, hypnosis can help improve their ability to cope.

I once had an eleven-year-old patient with chronic headaches who was a week away from undergoing neurosurgery to fix the presumed problem. This patient had been treated with many medications without relief and undergone extensive medical evaluations. The only abnormality identified was a minor brain malformation that usually causes no difficulties. However, since the headaches did not improve, the physician suggested the malformation could be the cause and recommended surgery. When I met this patient, I discovered that no psychological evaluation had been offered. I suggested postponing the surgery so that I could evaluate and treat for a possible psychological issue, and fortunately the neurosurgeon agreed. In just a few sessions, it became clear to me—and, more important, it became clear to this patient—that the troubles he was having weren't caused by unusual brain anatomy. The headache stemmed, in large part, from the patient finding it very difficult to deal with the academic pressures at his school. It ultimately resolved not with surgical intervention but after allowing the child to switch schools.

WHAT YOU CAN DO ON YOUR OWN

Listen closely and actively. Children want and deserve to be respected, and meeting this one simple need can help them feel empowered on multiple levels. By focusing on what your child is telling you and repeating it back so he or she can hear that you understand, you provide a number of positive affirmations. First, you give acknowledgment. It is part of human nature to want to be heard, and kids especially need this from their families because they may not always get it from teachers and friends. Second, you subtly encourage your child to think and speak independently. When you listen without steering or redirecting, you give children confidence in their ability to express themselves. Third, if your child has an environment where he or she can comfortably express fears or concerns, he or she may be less likely to bottle them up and allow them to manifest in other ways. The opportunity to talk through their troubles without feeling judged or directed can help kids make great strides in working through their own concerns and frustrations. Finally, as I have discovered, children often have a pretty good idea of what is bothering them. If you listen carefully, they may tell you exactly what needs to be addressed in order for them to heal.

THE POWER OF WORDS

5

Faith Healing?

How Words Alone Can Improve Health

Nearly every aspect of medicine has an artistic component as well as a scientific one, but this is rarely discussed because creativity and sensitivity are more difficult to observe, describe, measure, and replicate than pure science. That said, there's no way to understand hypnosis without looking at both the art and the science of it. A successful teacher of hypnosis must be able to utilize the power of words with empathy and creativity. He or she must be able to help patients relax and imagine realities that are different from what exists within the consultation room.

My first intense introduction to this concept occurred with Paul a year before I learned about hypnosis. At that time, Paul suffered from a severe allergic reaction and had to be resuscitated. This emergency intervention led to a lung collapse and the insertion of a chest tube.

The tube was removed once his lung healed, but Paul's mother called a week later to say her son was in agony. He had terrible pain at the site where the tube had been and was having trouble walking. She was worried he might have suffered brain damage during the resuscitation. This seemed like a big leap, but when I asked how she'd arrived at this suspicion, her answer was sobering.

"This wouldn't be the first time," she said. "It happened after a resuscitation when he was seven. He needed six months of rehab after that."

I notified the hospital to expect Paul for admission and contacted the neurologist and pain service to do assessments.

Paul was brought to the hospital in a wheelchair. During the first hours after admission, he underwent tests, including a brain scan and nerve-conduction study prescribed by the neurologists to identify why Paul couldn't walk. The nerve study was particularly uncomfortable, requiring that needles be inserted into Paul's forearm and electric currents run through them to measure how well his nerves were working. The pain specialist had little to offer for control of his chest pain.

That afternoon I went to see Paul, knowing there was no obvious physical explanation for his paralysis. He was sitting in the recliner beside his bed, so upset he was shaking. When I asked what was wrong, he glared.

"It *hurts!*" he said. "The needles in my arm hurt. My chest hurts. I can't walk!" His face twisted in sorrow and frustration, and he bowed his head. "I'm sick and tired of being sick," he added in anger. "I want to go home!"

I sat in front of him and asked him to look up. Making eye contact, I said, "You're going to be OK." I grasped his hands to steady the shaking. "You are going to get through this, just like you've gotten through all the other hard things in your life."

He was silent but listening.

"Once your pain goes away, you'll feel better," I continued, "and you'll be able to walk again."

He nodded slightly.

"I'll bet," I said, "that you'll be able to walk sooner than you think."

This earned me another glare, but it didn't seem to have the conviction I'd seen in the first one.

"You can relax," I said. "That can help you feel better."

As I was talking, his breathing slowed. His arms stopped trembling. And his glare turned into a fixed gaze that we shared.

Somehow the bond that formed at that moment prompted me to offer a suggestion. "How would you like to walk now?"

He started to shake his head but then nodded.

I got bolder. "OK, let me help you stand. Let's see how far you can walk."

Paul stood slowly with my assistance. When I suggested he take a step, he did it tentatively, grasping my shoulder. He was unsteady but remained upright. As he took one slow step after another, his confidence increased, and he loosened his grip on me. At the door, he lowered his arm, appearing to focus on putting one foot in front of the other. Within a few moments we were out of the room and slowly making our way down the brightly lit hallway.

"You're doing great!" I told him. "You're going to be just fine."

When we reached the end of the hall, we turned and walked at a faster pace back to Paul's room. When he sat back in the chair, his demeanor was changed. "I'm going to be all right," he said quietly. "I am going to be all right." By then he was well on his way to being able to go home.

Leaving the hospital that day, I replayed the incident over and over in my head: a boy with a long and complex medical history, who had already known more medical emergencies than most people experience in a lifetime, who could not walk one minute and was able to the next. I wondered, *Was this some kind of faith healing?*

THE WEIGHT OF A SUGGESTION

I know now that Paul's transformation that day is largely traceable to the potential for our statements and verbal affirmations to influence our experience: the power of words.

Successful hypnosis relies heavily on this power that we all experience but rarely think about. If you spend an hour with someone who complains incessantly and an hour with someone who speaks with purpose, hope, and good intentions, you can feel the difference as the words of negativity or positivity wash over you. This simple fact of language is one we experience intuitively and constantly and one that's been acknowledged for centuries. The biblical book of Proverbs says, "Pleasant words are like a honeycomb; Sweetness to the soul and health to the bones."[1] We're also told, "Death and life are in the power of the tongue."[2] In fact, at the beginning of the Bible, we learn that God created the entire world with His words.

Even though it's currently impossible to quantify the power of words over a lifetime, research is able to shed some light on how they impact us in the moment. Studies have demonstrated that simply hearing negative words raises subjects' levels of anxiety-inducing hormones and that even a single negative interjection can fire up the amygdala—the area frequently referred to as our brain's "fear center" for the way it controls emotional rather than logical responses. Notably, in a study in which children used different kinds of language to talk about themselves, when they engaged in negative self-talk, their anxiety levels went up. It seems it doesn't have to be other people's words that shape our realities—our own can do it as well.[3]

In studies investigating the power of positive words in particular, results are both thought provoking and promising. Just thinking and speaking positive words like *peace* and *hope* can strengthen our cognitive function and alter the way we approach questions and problems, causing us to lean more toward constructive action than emotional reaction. With a steady diet of positive language over time, these reactions become well-ingrained habits.[4]

Children are uniquely positioned to benefit or suffer from the power of words for a number of reasons. First, they tend to more readily embrace the fact that words can shape both perception and reality. This is why they love listening to stories. When they're young and still accustomed to learning through play, they frequently experiment with language, use their imaginations, and think outside convention. As teens, they are in a phase of rapid change, so they often readily adopt new ways of thinking (because they're already doing it all the time as part of the process of growing up). All the while, they are continually learning to understand, master, and utilize language effectively.

Children are especially susceptible to the power of words as a means of shaping their sense of identity. In each stage of development, their relationships with authority figures are shifting and changing, but in each phase the voices of those people have power (as do the voices of peers). Kids can easily internalize descriptors, particularly ones that suggest something about a part of the child's character rather than about his or her actions. When it comes to kids with chronic health issues, negative voices that focus on their dependence, on physical or mental weakness, or on an inability to do one thing or another can become defining as they develop their sense of self.

Conversely, positive input can help children manage chronic illness. An authority figure's suggestion that a child can master a challenge can serve as a foundation for a child's development of resilience. Contrast two parents' reactions to an eight-year-old with asthma who is complaining of shortness of breath. One concerned parent asks the child several questions in order to ensure that the child does not need to be rushed to the hospital and then administers an inhaler. The second parent suggests that the child use calming techniques and self-administer the inhaler, something the child has already been taught how to do. The first child learns to be dependent on the parent and perhaps develops anxiety when a parent is not around; the second child learns independence and resilience.

We adults, more set in our ways and reliant on expectations of how things *should* be, often have to make more of an effort to open ourselves to possibilities beyond what we've learned to expect. We often have to put more energy into learning how to listen and choose our words carefully than the young people around us.

THE PLACEBO EFFECT

Proof of the power of words and suggestion in medicine is readily available and supported through research on the placebo effect. Remarkably, in countless studies, patients given sugar pills or saline injections with the same appearance as medications and told those medications may help them *do* improve. In many cases, this holds true even when patients are informed that the pills are made up of inactive ingredients that have helped others. Studies have also demonstrated that active treatments are frequently less effective when they are given surreptitiously instead of announced and given where patients can see them.[5]

On the simplest level, we can see the placebo effect in tender loving care administered at home. When a parent lovingly offers a bowl of chicken soup or puts a bandage on an injury, a child feels comforted and perhaps even rallies from temporary illness or ailment. There is untold power in the words and intention of "This will make you feel better."

In some circles, once researchers demonstrate that improvement found in a study occurs equally in patients administered a drug or placebo, the main conclusion is that the drug should not be used for therapy. But such researchers fail to consider that the placebo effect provides evidence of the power of the human mind to heal. If placebos work, then somewhere in the depths of our minds we have the capacity to regulate affected systems and symptoms—and one of the catalysts of this power is the words we choose. If we know this is true, shouldn't we be working to better understand and implement it?

Early in my career as a pulmonologist, I told my patients' parents that over-the-counter (OTC) cough medicines don't work any better than placebos, a fact that's been demonstrated in numerous studies. Because of this and the potential for side effects, I recommended against using OTC medications for cough. Later I would realize my advice was incomplete, because even though OTC medications were not better than placebos, the placebo effect *did* help children with their coughs. The result had nothing to do with the efficacy of the medicine and everything to do with the mental and physical capacity to self-regulate. Later in my career, I began recommending that children be given something for the cough, such as teaspoonful of honey, because it can help them feel better even if there's no strictly physical or chemical basis for the improvement.

Hypnosis is one of the most fundamental and functional ways to tap into this tremendous but poorly understood power that children have within themselves. Like placebos, this therapy focuses largely on effecting change for symptoms that are managed by the brain—like pain, anxiety, fatigue, and nausea. All of these are sources of incalculable suffering that are entwined with the conditions that cause them. The benefits of managing these symptoms can be immeasurably powerful: easing the constant stomachache of a child with irritable bowel syndrome, relieving nausea for a child undergoing chemotherapy, or tamping down anxiety so a child can get a good night's sleep or go to school.

In each of these cases, the impact of therapy starts with words. They are one of the main tools I use to make children feel welcome in my office, to help them understand they are in control of the situation there, to guide them to a state of relaxation, and to encourage them to tap into their own power to manage how they feel. Each step relies on positive, empowering speech. The effect of words is augmented by how they are delivered, be it loudly, softly, rhythmically, or with long, interspersed pauses. Further, nonverbal communication can accentuate the power of words, such as an accompanying smile or gazing into a child's eyes. In later chapters we'll explore other, deeper mechanisms at work, but it's amazing what the power of positive words alone can accomplish for kids who are feeling frustrated, anxious, fearful, or depressed.

WHAT YOU CAN DO ON YOUR OWN

Utilizing the power of words to encourage and empower our children doesn't have to be (and shouldn't be) limited to therapy appointments. Utilize words at home to foster positive attitudes and outcomes.

Because the words we use hold significant sway over our thoughts and actions, I teach children and their parents to frame ideas in a positive way. A simple way of changing a negative statement into a positive framework is to start with "I wish . . ." or "I want . . ."

For example, instead of saying, "I am feeling badly," you can say, "I wish to feel better." When someone describes their bad feeling, the brain focuses on that thought, and the bad feeling is reinforced. By contrast, when the thought focuses on feeling better, the brain starts to think and act on a path to help achieve that goal.

Encourage your child by focusing on empowerment rather than just flattery. If your child receives an improved grade on a test, praise her for the commitment she made to studying or ask her how she studied to achieve that outcome. When children talk about actions they are taking, that helps them feel in control of their own fates. Every small step toward taking ownership of solutions to their problems is a step in the right direction.

When you're talking about goals, use "when" instead of "if." In this way you convey your confidence in your child's ability to accomplish something. "Try" is another word to avoid because it leaves room for failure. As Yoda said in *Star Wars*, "Do or do not. There is no try."

Weak and Strong, Heavy and Light

A Reason to Believe

We all know that perception has power, but we often underestimate just how forceful it can be. When I first meet patients, I want to impress upon them that their thoughts can create powerful change in their bodies. This serves a dual purpose: first, engaging and allying them with me to help improve their physical and mental health and, second, giving them a reason to believe in the potential that learning self-hypnosis might hold for them. One of the first experiences I share with new patients invites them to participate in a demonstration of this concept.

Just like any kind of exercise, hypnosis is more effective when the patient (and, in the case of pediatric patients, also the parent) believes in it. Think about the way you approach a workout regimen or the way a child studies for an exam. Going through the motions by rote, doing the minimum, and doubting you can succeed doesn't have nearly the impact of approaching the endeavor with commitment and confidence. A child's buy-in is critical to the success of hypnosis because he or she ultimately controls it. Because parents have such a strong influence on their children, their engagement is important too.

These exercises give my patients—sometimes for the first time—a sense that they have a profound influence over their own realities.

Children who see their own statements having weight are able to approach hypnosis (and many other activities) with confidence, thereby increasing their odds of achieving successful outcomes.

WEAK AND STRONG

After my first years of using hypnosis with patients and seeing how it was changing their lives, I began writing about their experiences in medical literature and lecturing to share my findings with other health care practitioners. As a result, colleagues began referring patients to me specifically for hypnotic intervention.

One of these patients was Joseph, who was exhibiting symptoms of vocal cord dysfunction that occurred during exercise while he was training for the ninth-grade cross-country season. His pediatrician had prescribed a number of asthma and allergy medications. Rather than refer him for further tests or surgery, Joseph's doctor sent him to be evaluated for hypnosis. I explained to him, as I do to every new patient, that hypnosis starts with recognizing the power of words. I offered to give him a demonstration. His mom could participate, too, if he wanted.

"This is a physical example," I said, "so please stand up and face me." We stood looking at each other.

"Are you right-handed or left-handed?" I asked.

"Right."

"OK, put out your arm like this," I instructed, extending my left arm so it was parallel to the floor and pointing to the side. Joseph mirrored me with his right arm.

"Now, your job is to keep your arm up as best you can, even when I press down on it."

He nodded.

"OK. Let's see how strong you are," I said as I placed my left hand over the middle of his arm. "Resist me as I press down." Joseph did exactly that, and I was unable to push down his arm.

"You're strong," I commented. "Good job."

"Now, we're going to do the same thing again, except this time you are going to say, 'I'm weak, I'm weak, I'm weak.' But don't let me push down your arm."

"Got it," he replied.

"Go ahead, say it," I prompted.

Joseph looked at me and said, "I'm weak, I'm weak, I'm weak." When I pressed his arm, it went down easily. He looked puzzled.

"Now we'll do the same thing again, except this time you're going to say, 'I'm strong, I'm strong, I'm strong.' OK?"

Joseph set his jaw and stared hard at his arm. "I'm strong, I'm strong, I'm strong."

When I pressed his arm, it didn't budge.

"How'd you do that?" I asked him.

"I'm not sure. Did you press harder when my arm went down?"

"Actually I pressed less because it went down so easily. How do you think that works?"

"I guess what I say makes my arm weak or strong?"

"That's exactly right," I answered. "What you say is what happens. That's a very important principle. So tell me, are you a positive self-talker or a negative one?"

"I'm pretty positive."

"And when you begin to run a race, what goes through your mind?"

"Oh," he said, "I worry that I may start having trouble breathing."

"And then you do have trouble," I concluded. "So, in a way, your words may have been contributing to your difficulties."

"I guess so," he said. "I need to be more positive."

"Exactly. Now let's try something different. What do you predict will happen if you say, 'I'm not weak, I'm not weak, I'm not weak?'"

"I think I'll be strong, but not quite as strong as when I say I am strong," he said.

"Let's try it."

"I'm not weak, I'm not weak, I'm not weak," he said. I pressed down on his arm, and it went down easily.

Joseph shrugged and looked at me.

"What happened?" I asked.

"I was weak?"

I nodded. "Why do you think?"

He thought about this a minute. "Was it because I used the word 'weak'?"

"That's right. Your mind focuses on the major word in the sentence, which is 'weak,' and ignores the 'not.' So when you're being positive with yourself, it's important that you use positive language, like 'I want to breathe well,' rather than a negative phrase like 'I'm not going to have a breathing problem.'"

"I get that," he said.

I added, "It's really important when you use positive talk that you tell yourself something that you believe fully. For example, if you start having trouble breathing, you should not tell yourself that your breathing is fine. Rather, you might tell yourself that you want your breathing to be easier, which you know is one hundred percent true."

Joseph nodded.

"Have a seat," I invited. "I want to give you a real-life example of the power of positive talk." Joseph leaned back on the couch, and I settled into my chair.

"One time, my friend Lois came from Boston to visit me in La Jolla," I started. "One of the big problems we have here is a lack of parking. I told Lois I'd take her to a restaurant, but I warned her it would be difficult to find parking.

"Lois told me, 'It won't be any problem. Wherever I go, there's always parking.'

"I didn't know what she meant, but I didn't think much about it until she came to visit and we went out to eat. Amazingly, there was parking everywhere, even in front of the restaurant. It was like she had parking karma."

Joseph smiled.

"Lois went back to Boston," I continued, "but I kept thinking about that moment. I wondered if positive talk was involved. I started telling myself 'I am going to find a space' everywhere I went. And it has worked. Apparently I have parking karma now too." I smiled in response to Joseph's raised eyebrows.

"It even works at our favorite beach, which only has a tiny parking lot. On a sunny Saturday, in the middle of the afternoon, I can tell my kids, 'Watch this, I am going to find parking'—and voilà—a space opens up in front of me."

"How does this work?" I asked Joseph. "Is it magic? Does positive talk make parking spots materialize? Actually, there is a scientific explanation for this and a nonscientific explanation. What do you think the scientific explanation is?"

Joseph thought for a moment. "Maybe you're more focused on finding parking spots, and that's why you see them."

"That's a good guess," I responded, "but it's unlikely, because when I look for parking, I always look closely."

"Maybe it's just a coincidence?" he offered.

"Also unlikely. If it were a coincidence, it wouldn't happen every time."

"I don't know how, then," he said.

"OK, I'll tell you. The scientific explanation goes like this: When I am positive, I become more patient. Since I know I am going to find a parking spot, if the parking spots are full, I will go around the block again to look for one. In the beach example, if I had been negative, I would have said to myself, 'The lot looks full, so I'll park somewhere else.' Instead, I drove right in and looked for a spot. So, by being positive I gave myself more chances."

Joseph smiled.

"But there is also a nonscientific explanation," I said. "You have to experience it for yourself in order to understand it. If you throw positivity into the universe, it comes back to you. When I am positive, I believe the universe sometimes brings me good fortune." I added, "The reverse also is true. When people are negative, the universe reflects back their negativity. This is why it's important to be positive—for me to be positive and for you to be positive too."

Joseph nodded and said, "OK."

"Sometimes people have a hard time with nonscientific explanations," I went on. "Science depends on things that can be observed and measured, but we can't do either of those things with our thoughts. That's why no one can *prove* that positive thoughts can influence the way the universe responds. But just because something cannot be studied scientifically does not mean it doesn't exist."

Joseph nodded. "I believe that," he said.

"Right!" I exclaimed. "Do you know who Henry Ford was?"

"Sure. He built the first car."

"Exactly," I affirmed. "Henry Ford also knew about the power of words and thoughts. He said, 'Whether you think you can or think you can't, you are right.'"

Joseph pondered this notion. "So," he said slowly, "if I think I can do something, this will help me do it?"

"Yup."

"This gives me a lot of ideas!" he said.

HEAVY AND LIGHT

I congratulated Joseph on how astutely he'd understood the power of his words. Next, I wanted to show him how the imagery associated with those words holds power as well.

"OK," I said. "Let's try something else. For this demonstration we'll need another volunteer."

I peered around the room as if there were plenty to choose from.

Joseph looked quizzically at me; then he turned to his mother, the only other person present, and gamely said, "How about this lady?"

"Perfect," I responded. "For this demonstration, you get to stand in the middle of the office facing me, and your mother will stand behind you."

Joseph and his mother followed the instructions. "Now," I continued, "your mother gets to pick you up."

"Pick him up?" she said doubtfully. Joseph was fairly big for his age.

"If you can!" I encouraged. She put her hands around his waist and lifted him about three inches off the ground. She groaned a bit, and Joseph laughed.

"Now I have a secret to tell Joseph," I said as I gestured for him to come closer to me. I whispered in his ear, "Imagine that your feet are glued to the ground and you have big lead weights tied to your ankles."

Joseph nodded and chuckled as he walked back over to his mother.

"Pick him up again," I instructed.

His mother groaned as she attempted to do so. But Joseph had become quite limp and cumbersome, and she was unable to lift him even an inch. When she let go and stepped back to look at him, he laughed out loud. She smiled—confused but willing to play along.

"I have another secret for you," I said. He stepped toward me and leaned in. "This time, imagine you have a belt tied around your waist, and there are thousands of helium balloons attached, pulling you into the air, just like in the movie *Up*."

Joseph grinned as he went back to his mother. "Please pick him up again," I instructed. This time, she easily lifted him six inches off the ground.

"He was lighter!?" she exclaimed.

"How did that work, Joseph?" I asked.

"It worked great," he exclaimed.

"I'll let you explain to your mom what you did," I said. "The important thing to understand about it is that what you imagine and the things you visualize have power, just like the things you say. Now if you're ready, it's time to learn how to put words and imagery together in hypnosis."

MAKING A SIGN

Since my earliest days of using hypnosis, I'd been learning how to better guide patients through the experience. It was clear that the more they understood the *why* of the things they were doing, the more invested they felt in the process. As I guided Joseph into a relaxed state for the first time, I explained each step. Like many children, he chose the beach for his relaxing place. Also like many younger children, he was quite capable of moving around and keeping his eyes open during hypnosis. Older children tend to stay very still and keep their eyes closed during this process, but that's not important to its success in some children. Joseph was a boy who didn't find it easy to sit still before we began hypnosis, and so I wasn't surprised to see him shuffling his feet and occasionally looking around the room while he was doing it.

I asked Joseph to describe what he was experiencing using each of his senses. I explained that he was aiming to achieve relaxation that involved as much of his brain as possible.

"The more you imagine your senses, the more real the experience will seem, and the more relaxed you can become," I told him. "If we scanned your brain while you imagined with your senses, each time you conjured a different sense, a different part of your brain would become involved."

Joseph smiled at this idea and described the way the sun felt on his shoulders and the sand felt on his toes. He told me he could hear seagulls squawking and see waves rolling up onto the beach. He said that he could taste chocolate ice cream and that he was playing Frisbee with a friend.

Clearly this was a child with a vivid imagination—a promising indicator that he would become good at self-hypnosis.

After working with dozens of children, I'd adopted a routine next step in cases like Joseph's: encouraging children to learn to associate a gesture they can control with the relaxed feeling they have in hypnosis. This is an especially valuable tool for kids for whom anxiety plays a role—those with breathing issues such VCD or asthma or with headaches, stomachaches, and even school-related stress.

"Now you have an important job," I said. "You get to pick your own personal relaxation sign. This is a signal you can use whenever you want to calm yourself, even when you are not doing hypnosis. You could make a very visible sign, like this," I said, raising my hands above my head and then slowly lowering them in front of my chest. "But then people might wonder what the heck you're doing."

He smiled at this but remained quiet.

"Instead of doing something big, I recommend picking a subtle gesture, like making a fist, or thumbs-up, or crossing your fingers." I showed him these alternatives with my right hand.

With his right hand, Joseph made a tight fist and lifted it to show me.

"That's perfect," I said. "From now on, whenever you make that fist, you'll be able to relax just like in hypnosis. This will help with your breathing. If you feel like your throat could get tight, make your sign and notice that your breathing can remain steady and easy. If you develop breathing problems, you can just relax with your sign and your breathing will improve immediately. You can use it anytime, even before you have symptoms. In fact, that's the best time—that can prevent the breathing problem from starting in the first place."

Joseph nodded, clenching and unclenching his fist.

Giving children a gesture to associate with the way they feel in hypnosis becomes a sort of a shortcut to a psychological and physical state. With just a few sessions of practice at home, Joseph would learn to calm his mind and his breathing at will by using this tool. He would be able to achieve this almost instantly, rather than having to work his way through the steps to "full" hypnosis to get there. Just as most people can relate to feeling affirmative when they give a thumbs-up or hopeful when they cross their fingers, Joseph would feel relaxed when he made this fist. Creating this powerful association between a simple act of the body and what the mind perceives is called *anchoring*, an apt name for a gesture that can help kids feel centered and calm in moments when they might otherwise feel overwhelmed or adrift.

A STATE OUT OF TIME

"Once you rehearse your relaxation sign you can spend as much time in hypnosis as you'd like," I continued. "You can imagine being on the beach for a minute, an hour, a month, or a year. Time has no meaning when you are in hypnosis."

"How does that work?" he asked.

"In hypnosis, you can focus on the imagery and ideas that are deep within your mind. When those thoughts do not include paying attention to clock time, you can lose track of it. Have you ever read a book and became so interested in it that you didn't realize how long you had been reading?"

Joseph nodded.

"It's like that. In our daily lives, we rarely have the opportunity to choose how we perceive the passage of time, but we do have moments when we take a step back from it, when we are engaged with it in a different way. Hypnosis allows us to do that. That's why you can go to your relaxing place for just a few minutes and come back as calm as if you'd had the whole morning to unwind."

By the time Joseph and his mom left my office after that first appointment, we were all confident hypnosis was going to help him control his VCD. He had wholeheartedly embraced the process, and that engagement would be key to his practice routine and ultimately to his success.

WHAT YOU CAN DO ON YOUR OWN

Guided imagery is not the exclusive province of any specific therapy. You can encourage and prompt your child to think of a favorite place, real or imagined, and ask questions or converse about what the child experiences there. This kind of exercise can start as something simple and fun at the dinner table, on a car ride, or at bedtime—imagining or reliving the sights, sounds, smells, tastes, and tactile sensations of a special place. However, engaging in this kind of imagery is more than just a game. It allows your child to strengthen his or her ability to pull back from one environment and plug into another at will.

Many children participating in this kind of exercise are just discovering that the way they feel in the moment is not solely dictated by outside circumstances. Being able to envision and consciously choose to focus on a calm, positive, safe environment is an empowering skill they can apply in all areas of their lives. For example, children can be taught to take a moment to calm themselves by imagining their special place before they start taking a big test in school or participating in a high-stakes athletic competition. Their subsequent improved performances can serve as motivation for ongoing use of self-regulation skills.

The Red Headache

Safe, Effective, Age-Appropriate Pain Management

Almost every physician spends a substantial portion of his or her time trying to categorize, pinpoint the origin of, and provide relief from pain. We work to understand its mechanisms and gain any advantage over it for our patients. Some of us devote entire careers to studying pain's many forms, among them sharp or dull, acute or chronic, severe or mild, localized or general, and rooted in physical and/or psychological causes. Sometimes pain is a mystery unto itself, and sometimes it's a critical diagnostic clue. Many doctors consider it as much a vital sign as temperature or blood pressure, but it's not one we can precisely measure with a thermometer or a cuff. Instead, we must rely on subtle cues and each child's own reporting.

Complicating matters is the fact that emotional and psychological factors routinely hold sway over the way pain presents, how it's perceived, and how it's communicated to peers, parents, and medical professionals. Most of us have encountered situations in which this is obvious: A child tells friends he's fine but cries when he sees his mother. An athlete follows through on a play after a collision but collapses with an injury off the field. A preschooler who is actively engaged in play appears to have forgotten a stomachache that was intolerable just moments before.

Some pain seems beyond the patient's ability to influence, but much of it is not—a hint that a part of us has the capacity to regulate our pain experience.

Despite its sometimes enigmatic nature, pain is the single most studied area in which hypnosis has been proven to be an effective therapeutic tool. Hypnosis has been investigated and validated as treatment for pain from headaches, medical procedures, cancer treatment, irritable bowel syndrome, pulmonary disease (which often causes chest pain), and burn treatment.[1] It is unequivocally proven to be useful in alleviating varieties of pain, and unlike other leading forms of treatment, it can be directly controlled by the patient without potentially harmful side effects. People don't become addicted to hypnosis or overdose on it. No one has ever developed a physical ailment as a result of using it too much. Instead, patients who successfully learn to control their pain through hypnosis often report feeling calmer, more confident, and more hopeful—effects we all welcome.

AN OVERLOOKED SOLUTION

In my own practice, I see patients who are dealing with pain almost every day. Sometimes we know what the problem is: complications of cancer, cystic fibrosis, inflammatory bowel disease, sickle cell crises, or perhaps joint inflammation caused by juvenile arthritis. Children with these and other chronic conditions may be seeking to change or expand the pain management options in their toolboxes, often because something in their current regimen isn't practical or sufficient.

The root cause of the pain may remain unknown, even after the child, family, and clinicians have worked diligently to uncover it. Kids with chronic stomachaches, for example, are often subjected to a this-will-pass phase, trips to the pediatrician, then a specialist, imaging studies or endoscopy, and dietary changes (with or without the introduction of antacids or pain medications) before hypnosis is considered. Kids with severe headaches that recur or persist over months and even years may have endured escalating regimens of tests and prescriptions. When no other label fits, many of these children are diagnosed with *functional pain*—a blanket term to describe pain with no known organic origin.

All children experience pain at some point in childhood, but when it persists or worsens—regardless of the reason—it can result in absences from school, the inability to participate in sports and other activities, expensive and sometimes invasive investigations, and stress for both child and family.

Given the proven record of hypnosis to reduce or alleviate many different kinds of pain, that it is so seldom being recommended as a front-line therapy, instead of a last-ditch effort when everything else has failed, seems like a terrible oversight. I have worked with thousands of children who have learned to better manage their pain through hypnosis. For some, it turns out to be a viable therapy that fills in the gaps of an existing regimen. For others, it is a solution to the pain problem. This was the case for Rich, a preteen who came to my office after hurting every day for months.

WHAT COLOR IS YOUR PAIN?

Rich developed a headache on his twelfth birthday, one intense enough to bring his celebration to an end and send him to bed before dark. He felt better in the morning, but by early afternoon the sharp pain in his forehead had returned. The next day brought the same pattern, and so did the day after that. Days turned into weeks and then months, and the headache returned. Rich started to dread the pain he knew was coming each day, and some days he was too uncomfortable to eat. On other days, he struggled to do his homework or enjoy activities with his family. His parents worried something serious might be wrong.

Rich was evaluated by his pediatrician, a neurologist, and an otolaryngologist, but no one was able to identify a cause of the unrelenting headache.

When Rich had suffered through six months of daily headaches with no improvement, his pediatrician decided to try a different tack. She referred him to me.

That first afternoon, I asked Rich to describe his pain.

"I hate it," he said. "It's like it never goes away. It feels kind of like something is pushing on my skull from the inside. When it gets bad, I can't think about anything else."

I asked him to rate the intensity of his pain on a zero-to-ten scale, with a zero meaning no headache and ten meaning the worst headache he could imagine. He said it was a seven that afternoon but often got worse as the day wore on, sometimes even reaching a nine or ten.

We talked about hypnosis and the power of words and imagery, and when I asked whether he'd like to try using it to help control his pain, Rich was eager.

As we worked through the steps of Rich getting comfortable, breathing deeply, and relaxing his muscles from head to toe, he said the level of his headache stayed the same.

When I asked him to describe the place where he felt the most relaxed and content, he said it was Disneyland. (I find it a little ironic that the places many children choose for relaxation are anything but for adults.) He described it in great detail, right down to the "old-time" music he heard, the fresh-baked cookies he smelled, and the bricks he felt underfoot on Main Street.

"You're doing a great job," I said. "Now let's use your imagination to focus on helping your head feel better."

"OK."

"Please look around and find a mirror. Take your time and let me know when you locate it."

A moment later, Rich announced he had found one.

"Great," I said. "Now look into the mirror. It's a special one. It colors your body the way that you feel. I'd like you to look at the reflection of your forehead. What color do you see there?"

Rich frowned at the subtle reminder of his headache and answered, "It's red."

"All right," I continued. "That color shows what your head looks like when it hurts. What color do you think the mirror will show you once your head feels better?"

"Blue!"

"Great. Now watch the mirror. Let's change the color. Your head is slowly changing from that angry red to purple to a soothing blue. As it's happening, notice what happens to the comfort level in your head."

Rich's forehead wrinkled a bit as he focused.

"It's gone blue," he said quietly, confirming he could visualize the transition.

"And what number is your pain right now?"

"It's down to a five or six."

"That's good," I said, encouraged that he'd seen a little improvement. "You're doing a great job!"

Rich opened his eyes, looked at me, and smiled slightly.

"OK," I said. "Let's try another way to improve how your head feels."

I thought for a moment, channeling other conversations and sessions I'd had with kids his age to come up with another effective image. I knew of one that always caught their interest. "If a creature were causing your headache," I asked, "what would it be?"

Rich looked quizzically at me.

"Use your imagination," I encouraged him.

He closed his eyes and mulled it over before answering, "It's a woodpecker."

"What's it doing?" I asked.

"Pecking at my head. Pecking a hole in my head."

"OK. Think about what the woodpecker likes. Is there something it would rather be doing instead of bothering your head?"

"Pecking at a tree?" Rich said.

"Of course. So, why don't you imagine a beautiful, tall tree with lots of branches standing twenty feet away from you? Now show it to the woodpecker and tell it to go. Once it flies over there, notice how your head feels differently."

He paused for a moment. "It flew to the tree. It's pounding on it with its beak. And my head feels better."

"What number is your pain?" I asked.

"Three."

I told him that was wonderful, that he was doing a great job, and then decided to try a third technique. "Let's do one more thing," I said, "one more way to get your head to feel better. Could you go back to Disneyland and find a ride called 'Rich's Mansion'? You'll know it's your ride because there will be a big sign right over it with your name."

Rich was quick to go along with this suggestion, and in a matter of seconds he announced that he'd found the ride.

"Now, go in and notice that your mansion has a lot of rooms," I said. "Each room is labeled with one of your body parts. You might see the stomach room, the leg room, the hand room. . . . Find the one that's labeled 'head room.'"

"OK," he said. "I found it."

"Good. Now go inside and look at the panels that control everything in your head, like how it moves, how you're thinking, and how you're feeling. I'd like you to find the panel that controls your head's comfort level."

"Got it!" he said.

"Perfect. Now some people see buttons, some people see dials, and some people see levers. What do you see?"

"A lever."

"What do you think happens when you lower the lever?"

"I feel better?"

"Exactly. So lower the lever slowly and notice what changes."

Rich appeared focused, and then he opened his eyes. "My headache is gone," he said. "Totally gone!"

I told him that was wonderful and that he should go home and practice hypnosis every day so he could learn to be calm and in control. "You can get good at this," I said, "and if you need to, you can use any of the skills I taught you to make your head feel comfortable."

TOOLS OF THE TRADE

Assigning color, introducing an animal to represent an antagonist that can be redirected, visualizing a tiny version of oneself inspecting the inside of the body, and creating a power control for pain are among dozens of analogies and metaphors clinicians can utilize to help children engage with and feel control over pain. It's easy to think that these things are just games, but for the child in hypnosis, the scenarios are working tools. By guiding Rich to find three different ways to visualize and reduce his pain under his own power, I hoped he would be able to choose at least one that he would feel comfortable practicing and could succeed with at home.

All but the youngest children tend to respond well to imagining a mechanical control for their pain. After establishing the child's pain level on a scale at the start of a session, we can compare how he or she perceives pain while implementing a tool—a switch, a turning or sliding dial, a mute button, or something similar—by subsequently rechecking with the same zero-to-ten scale.

The analogies we use in hypnosis therapy vary depending on the age, symptom, and perception of the child. One professional key for any clinician using hypnosis is learning to think up suggestions on the spot, utilizing imagery offered by the children themselves. Imagery constructed by the clinician may feel less relevant to a child or, in worst-case scenarios, can actually worsen a child's symptoms. For example, a clinician who offers a calming beach scene may induce a terrified reaction in a child who has experienced a near-drowning episode. Thus, the most therapeutic images are the ones the kids play a role in concocting. The more they are involved in the process, the safer they can feel and the more empowered they become when they achieve the desired result.

ADAPTING TO ANY AGE

Very young children aren't able to understand and follow if-then directions, so they require more age-appropriate guidance to accomplish pain control. Fortunately, they are also highly imaginative and open to creative suggestions that distract them, refocus their attention, and help give them perspective. This is especially important because little kids frequently jumble their emotions, so anxiety and fear can easily be interpreted as pain. Most of us do this to some extent, but young children do it exceptionally well—as any parent can attest who's ever seen a child recoil, as if in pain, at the sight of a needle.

For kids under five, an alternate method is to engage them in storytelling that incorporates a pain-lowering mechanism. For example, I treated a four-year-old girl who was referred because of anxiety and pain relating to uncomfortable daily bandage changes. Sally's discomfort was the result of a rare condition that causes skin to blister or peel at the merest touch. It's been described as causing children's skin to be as delicate as butterfly wings.

In order to protect her skin, Sally required bandaging from neck to toes throughout her childhood—a process that was painful but necessary to protect her from injury and infection.

Looking for a way to create a metaphor she might be able to embrace, I inquired about her favorite story.

"Belle," she replied.

"From *Beauty and the Beast*?" I asked.

She nodded. I was glad this was a story I knew (and over the years I've developed a passing knowledge of lots of children's books, movies, and television shows through this process). If the story had been one I didn't know, though, I would have asked Sally to tell me about it.

"That's a great story," I said. "Do you remember when the light shines on the Beast at the end? What happens then?"

"He turns into a prince," she said.

"That's right. So, all you need to do when your bandages are changed is imagine Belle shining a light on you. What will happen?"

"I'll be a princess?" she smiled.

"That's right!"

The next morning, when her bandages were changed, Sally cried and became upset as usual. Her parents asked if she had used her imagination as I had taught her. She told them that she couldn't because she didn't have her Belle doll. This was unsurprising, as four-year-olds tend to respond best to the use of concrete objects rather than imagined ones.

The following day they reintroduced the story, Sally held her doll, and the bandages were changed without fuss. By having a hand in choosing the story, embracing it as something she could believe in, and even augmenting her ownership of it by determining it couldn't work without her doll, Sally was able to block the pain of her bandage changes and continue to do so daily.

This simple hypnotic guidance was effective for over two years. As children grow and mature, though, their pain-management needs change, too.

The next time I saw Sally, she was coming up on her seventh birthday, and the doll technique had stopped working. At that point, I offered her a "magic" rock "from the Black Forest near Belle's house." I explained that when she held the rock, its power would help make her more comfortable during the bandaging.

I keep a collection of rocks, seashells, and marbles in my office for occasions like this. Early elementary school–aged children often embrace the idea of having a talisman they can hold or have in their pocket, especially one they can believe has special powers to block, relieve, or erase discomfort.

Another two years passed before I saw Sally again—when the rock had lost its magic power for her. At that point, I taught her about her own "powers." I explained how she could cause her arms to levitate seemingly on their own by imagining that she was holding strings to many balloons or make herself heavy just by thinking about it—exercises I'd done with Joseph and countless other patients. Because she was older, I added an element of focus on Sally's special ability to make those things happen. I suggested that Sally could use her abilities to feel good during the bandage changes, and again she succeeded in feeling more comfortable.

These common hypnotic phenomena are all achievable by children and provide them with evidence of their own capabilities. I knew as Sally left that day that by the next time I saw her, she would be intellectually ready for more traditional hypnosis and, with it, she would learn to self-manage her pain for a long time to come.

To be effective, hypnotic suggestions must grow and change with the child, so clinicians who use hypnosis must make adjustments to match each patient's stage of development and individual concerns. Most important, regardless of the patient's age, his or her participation in creating the pain-management tool is critical to its success. The clinician doesn't influence the comfort-control technique or the color wheel; the child does.

For kids like Rich and Sally and thousands of others who find pain reduction and relief through hypnosis, one might wonder why such a painless, inexpensive, proven treatment wasn't introduced during the first weeks of discomfort rather than after months of trudging through ineffective investigations and interventions. One reason is that clinicians are concerned that use of hypnosis might mask a pain that indicates physical problems that need to be treated medically. While there is some merit to this concern, by the end of their initial evaluation, experienced clinicians typically have a good sense of whether pain is of physical origin. Furthermore, even when medications alleviate pain, that treatment can mask a physical problem that needs additional therapy. Thus, in the treatment of painful conditions, I believe clinicians must always be on the lookout for situations in which pain reduction through medication *or* hypnosis may be only part of appropriate medical management.

WHAT YOU CAN DO ON YOUR OWN

The simple act of rating their pain helps kids begin to think of it as something that is variable. If your child experiences passing headaches, stomachaches, or other body pains, or if he or she is dealing with chronic pain for a diagnosed condition, ask the child to use the zero-to-ten scale to assess its intensity. Even without hypnosis, you can then ask your child to participate in lowering that level. You might ask whether the child thinks medication, a warm bath, a cup of cocoa, or a game of cards might help. If you're confident that medication or any other form of intervention is necessary, suggest it as ancillary to your child's choice. The more you can follow his or her lead, the more your child will feel ownership of pain control when another pain intensity rating demonstrates improvement. Over the course of this process, you'll be helping your child feel that pain can be managed—that he or she is not simply a victim of it.

Bruce, the Boy with Seizures

Applying Hypnosis in Novel Ways

One of the most medically fascinating patients of my career was a six-year-old boy named Bruce. He initially came to me for treatment of his asthma, but it was impossible to separate the asthma from the host of other medical problems with which he was living. Bruce had a peanut allergy, an allergy to dust that caused his nose to run much of the time, acid reflux from his stomach, frequent ear infections, migraine headaches, and a seizure disorder that started when he had bleeding in his brain as a baby. He also sometimes developed fevers that lasted for weeks at a time without any known cause. One possibility was that the fevers were caused by his injured brain's inability to control his body temperature. Each of these health issues challenged Bruce and his family. Together they were a complicated, discouraging jumble of ailments.

Over the course of a year, we addressed these problems one at a time. After some trial and error, his asthma, allergy symptoms, and acid reflux were much improved. This progress was overshadowed, though, when Bruce began experiencing more frequent seizures. His mother reported that he was having an average of one each week, despite the antiseizure medications he was taking.

Typically, Bruce's seizures would start in the right side of his head, where he'd had the brain bleed. At first his eyes would turn to the left and his left hand would turn palm down. As long as the seizure stayed on the right side of his brain, Bruce was able to speak to his mother, tell her he was having an episode, and move the right side of his body. About three-quarters of the time, however, the seizure would spread to the left side of his brain. When this happened, his whole body would shake, and he'd lose the ability to speak. This was a cruel affliction for such a young child and a heartbreaking one for his family to have to watch without being able to help.

Some basic brain information: The brain conducts its business through electrical activity. An epileptic seizure is caused in the brain by uncontrolled activity (or "a storm") that can start because one nerve cell acts up. The right side of the brain controls the left side of the body, and the left side of the brain controls the right side of the body. The speech center in the brain is located on the left side, which is why Bruce could not talk when the seizure spread to the left side of his brain.

One reason Bruce's seizures didn't always spread throughout his brain was rooted in the damage he'd suffered as a child during his bleeding episode. It had included injury to the nerves that connect the two sides of the brain to each other (known as the corpus collosum). Those damaged connectors did not always conduct electrical activity from one side of Bruce's brain to the other. It was an unusual circumstance. Ironically, it was also the silver lining that allowed him to sometimes remain functional during a seizure.

BUFFERING THE STORM

Bruce's seizure disorder weighed on me. We'd made a great deal of progress with his other health issues, and I wondered whether I could help him with his remaining serious condition. I had been learning how hypnosis could help in many different health situations and started thinking about whether it could help prevent seizures. I knew that dogs could be trained to sense when their owners were about to have a seizure, which allowed the owners to take precautions before they became unable to control their bodies. My interpretation was that recognizable neurological changes must take place before a seizure starts. Suppose, I reasoned, that with use of hypnosis patients could be taught to think differently in a way that changed their brain activity when they first had warning of an impending seizure. Could that prevent a seizure from occurring?

Since Bruce sometimes was able to tell his mother that a seizure was starting, I thought that he could be a candidate for using hypnosis to prevent the problem from spreading. It was an unconventional thought and perhaps a long shot, but it wasn't impossible.

I broached the subject with Bruce's mother, telling her I thought there was a small chance Bruce could learn to prevent his seizures from spreading from the right to left side of the brain. I presented it as an experiment (which it was) and was careful not to create false hope for an unlikely cure, emphasizing instead that there was no potential downside to trying. At worst, Bruce's existing symptoms would continue. At best, we might see a measure of improvement.

Bruce's mom was happy to let me try to help. Next I took the idea to the little boy who had already endured more medical incidents and interventions in his young life than many people do over their lifetimes. Despite the restrictions and regimens his health issues foisted into his life, he had an adventurous spirit, and he was eager to do something new.

Rather than using a formal ritual, the process of entering hypnosis with younger kids often involves telling a story or engaging their imaginations with a pretend activity such as interacting with a superhero or transforming into royalty (as in Sally's bandaging case in chapter 7). The common objective of hypnosis in both older and younger children is learning how to change their mind-set in the hope that this will allow for a change in their symptoms.

Patients of all ages are most empowered in hypnosis when they utilize imagery with which they are familiar. For example, a child who is prompted to imagine how she would feel if her hands contained giant magnets would have no idea how to respond if she'd never played with magnets. The best way to find a useful framework of imagery is to go straight to the source: the child.

I asked Bruce what cartoon character he liked best, and he exclaimed, "SpongeBob SquarePants!"

Ah, SpongeBob. Even though I dislike his show, he has helped me treat a number of his young fans in my office.

"Great!" I said. "Did you know that when you have a seizure in one part of your brain, it's like a storm in your brain that scares it? Sometimes, the storm then travels to the other parts of your brain and scares them too."

Bruce looked wide-eyed at me, and I explained this again, gesturing from the right to the left side of my own head to explain the transfer.

"Do you know what SpongeBob is made out of?" I asked.

"Uh, yeah. A sponge."

"That's right. And what does a sponge have in it?"

"Holes?"

"That's right. So when you feel a storm coming, you can put Sponge-Bob on top of your head and let the storm pass through his holes. When you do that, the storm will blow away instead of scaring your brain. If you want, you can even put SpongeBob on at night so you will be safe from any storms."

The fact is, setting up an entire hypnotic intervention in a young child can take just a few minutes. The key is to create a metaphor that makes sense to the child. I suggested to Bruce's mother that she remind him about SpongeBob whenever a seizure started.

After his visit and with his parents' help, Bruce started putting his soft SpongeBob toy on his head every night and telling himself that if a storm came, it would pass through the holes in the sponge instead of his brain. In the weeks that followed, he transitioned from the actual toy to an imaginary version that he secured to his head with an imaginary chin strap several times each night at bedtime. Occasionally he'd say the strap wasn't on correctly or the imaginary SpongeBob was out of place, and he'd start his routine again—exercising a healthy amount of control over his own unique form of treatment.

Four months later, when I saw Bruce in clinic, he and his mother reported that he hadn't experienced a single seizure since his last appointment. The migraine headaches they had triggered were gone as well. He continued his nightly SpongeBob routine for the next several years. During this time, we worked through his other health issues, but he never had another seizure—even though his electroencephalogram (EEG), which measures brain electrical activity, remained abnormal.

How is this possible? Even after all these years, I don't fully understand the reach of hypnosis in the human mind, but in Bruce's case the most likely explanation hinges on his symptoms becoming functional over time. Here was a child who'd had seizures for much of his life. They were an affliction initially caused by a physical circumstance (most likely the brain bleed), but at some point they might have become a habit of the body rather than a necessary reaction to an organic stimulus.[1] In a million years, Bruce could not have faked the seizures that impacted every aspect of his life, but it turned out that he was able to undo this physical habit and stop manifesting these events in such a stressful, potentially dangerous way. The EEGs of some patients— pediatric and adult—indicate seizure activity when there are no obvious physical signs they are happening. Deep in Bruce's mind, he had tapped the capacity to join this symptomless group.

A second plausible theory is that Bruce was able to use hypnotic activity to create a disconnect between a stimulus (in this case, the flurry of activity on the right side of his brain) and a response (spreading of the abnormal electrical activity to the left side of his brain with resulting full-body seizures). In this patient who had a known disconnect between the left and right sides of his brain as a result of previous trauma, learning how to use that anomaly to his advantage would be a fitting resolution to his seizure disorder.

Months later, Bruce demonstrated yet another ability to control his mind with hypnosis. Even when his seizures had stopped, he continued to develop frequent high fevers, without an obvious physical cause.

"Does SpongeBob have a friend?" I asked him at a subsequent visit.

"Yeah!" he responded enthusiastically. "Patrick."

"I have an idea for you. Next time you have a fever, tell Patrick to turn on the air conditioning."

"OK! I can do that."

Three months later, Ben's mother reported that he continued to develop fevers, although they did not last as long as previously.

"Tell Patrick to keep the air conditioning on all of the time," I suggested.

Bruce no longer developed recurrent fevers after that visit. Somehow, the hypnotic suggestion had helped adjust his brain's ability to control his body temperature.

PLUMBING THE DEPTHS

Ample research indicates that, through the power of hypnosis, the human mind is capable of controlling systems we tend to think of as self-regulating. Studies have found that subjects can influence their body temperature, blood flow, pain perception, and, yes, seizure activity.[2] A growing body of evidence tells us that use of hypnosis can be a valuable contribution to the diagnosis of nonepileptic seizures—those not caused by abnormal brain wave activity.[3] It often takes EEG monitoring to determine whether epilepsy has caused a seizure since seizures in any form can be equally sudden, uncomfortable, and disruptive. Complicating matters, a single patient can have either or both kinds of seizures. In Bruce's case, the resolution of his physical seizures may indicate that they had been nonepileptic or that, in his case, hypnosis blocked the effects of epileptic seizures seen on his EEG.

I believe we have barely begun to understand the full impact pediatric patients can have on themselves when they embrace hypnosis and learn to use it. I have worked with patients with profound loss of function due to disease and chronic conditions who have directly benefited from managing their symptoms in this way.

Daniel, a twenty-one-year-old college student with severe total body weakness caused by spinal muscular atrophy, depended on a ventilator to breathe. He developed pneumonia, for which he required weeks of antibiotic therapy, aggressive chest physiotherapy, and inhalation therapy. Daniel learned hypnosis to relieve his anxiety during this acute illness, using imagery of going down a staircase to a beautiful park. Notably, when he imagined himself on the third step of the staircase, the pressure required to ventilate his lungs decreased by nearly half. After fifteen minutes of hypnosis, his blood oxygen level had risen by 30 percent. Following each hypnosis session, his ventilator pressure and oxygen level remained at their improved levels for hours.[4]

Daniel reported feeling much better after using hypnosis, and because his family and I could objectively monitor these levels while he was doing it, we could see that this improvement was far more than a psychological tool. Daniel was, in fact, breathing better, and his body was, in fact, benefiting from having more oxygen. When he learned he was able to make this difference under his own power, Daniel embraced hypnosis as the one medical intervention that caused him no physical discomfort or anxiety. He was eager to learn how he could use it in other ways.

As in Bruce's case, Daniel's hypnosis raises questions about the why and how of his improvement. It is possible that the enhancement of his lung function was the result of hypnosis-induced relaxation that led his chest-wall muscles to yield more readily to the ventilator-exerted pressure. It's also possible hypnosis led to improvement of his neuromuscular coordination, which in turn caused more efficient functioning of his respiratory system.

The mechanism behind each of these remarkable cases still requires investigation, but the results are promising. More important, each serves as a reminder that the potential benefits of hypnosis are only partially understood. Knowing this, it is reasonable to apply hypnosis in many situations in which the brain may be involved in manifesting symptoms. This is not a substitute for thorough medical evaluation and therapy, but it is a potentially valuable diagnostic tool and adjunct therapy.

I believe the attitude of the patient and clinician delving into this kind of murky territory should be playful and flexible, as in *Let's see what happens when we do this.* A clinician employing hypnosis with positivity and sensitivity can ensure his or her patient feels empowered by its use rather than let down if it does not help with a specific issue.

With each passing decade (and sometimes year to year), our medical and scientific communities become more empowered by technological and biological advances to understand exactly why cases like Bruce's and Daniel's improved with hypnosis. One day I believe we will have a clearer picture of the mechanics of these improvements, but until then we can be certain of one thing: these children's lives are better as a result of this unique therapy.

WHAT YOU CAN DO ON YOUR OWN

Assessing a child's health and making treatment recommendations is the province of the medical team, but anyone can engage in the welcome connections forged over a shared cultural touchpoint like a favorite book or film character. For young children, this can be productive on another level. It can be a short leap from talking about characters and the traits that make them special to the children themselves modeling those traits in their own way. You can encourage this behavior and make it an exercise in empowerment by actively reading or watching movies with your child and pointing out shared desirable characteristics. In Bruce's treatment, we focused on the fact that SpongeBob is, well, a sponge, but the trait that drew the child to the character in the first place might have been his optimism. Huckleberry Finn might be an example of resourcefulness, Harry Potter of resilience, and Katniss Everdeen of courage. Gently remind your child of his or her own strengths when their favorite characters demonstrate such strengths in action.

Storytelling is a time-honored method of teaching children how to work out life challenges. When we tell our children scary fairy tales, this allows them to express and work out their fears. When we tell them stories about heroes and dreams, children learn how to engage their imaginations in ways that strengthen them. With young children, I often tell stories that embed hypnotic suggestions for change.[5] Sometimes I make up a story on the spot, and at other times I retell an old favorite. Sharing a hopeful story about a child who is struggling with the same issues as your child can help him or her learn how to cope better.

9

What Would the Coach Say?

Using Hypnosis to Tap Inner Knowledge

Leo, a lanky fourteen-year-old and a nationally ranked basketball player, was referred to me by his pediatrician for obsessive-compulsive tendencies and relentless anxiety in his day-to-day life. Both conditions seemed to worsen after Leo experienced a concussion. When I met him, he was socially paralyzed by his psychological issues—unable to answer questions in class for fear of being wrong, unable to speak with his peers for fear of sounding foolish, unable to fulfill his role on the basketball team for fear of taking a wrong step or missing a shot. He worried constantly about whether he was smart enough, strong enough, and handsome enough and about whether he was likeable. His grades and basketball performance were suffering, and his parents reported that his insecurities and anxiety were impacting his sleep schedule and diet as well.

As a pediatrician, I see far too many young patients who suffer this kind of anxiety. In fact, as many as 30 percent of our children and teens grapple with anxiety disorders at some point.[1] Meeting these patients is always a sobering reminder that the psychological issues children face are devastatingly real and, if left unaddressed, may lead to lifelong consequences. Leo was a young man who might realistically earn a full athletic scholarship to a top university if he could learn to overcome the obsessive-compulsive behaviors and anxieties that were holding him back.

At his first appointment, he described the intrusive negative thoughts that dominated his mind. The cycle of self-doubt he was living in had become so severe that when he heard about other people's problems, he'd begin worrying he might have them as well. The most alarming of these was a peer who frequently talked about self-harm. Even though my patient had not done anything to harm himself, he'd internalized this obsessive concern and worried that one day he might.

In children, anxiety reveals itself in multifaceted ways. It serves as a direct detriment to healthy functioning in everyday life, which is the most pressing concern when families seek help. It also holds them back at a critical juncture. They fall short at a time when they should be exploring and developing their talents, learning that practice and commitment yield results, and beginning to envision life goals and how to achieve them.

I informed Leo that I was confident he could learn to better manage his anxiety. The explanation was simple to understand (though it would require work to implement). In a nutshell, anxiety is related to mindset. Often it's caused by a cycle that quickly ramps kids up from slightly edgy to borderline meltdown in predictable patterns. The patient thinks about something going wrong; then, when it does go wrong, he or she dwells on the failure and becomes more anxious. Leo had been in this mind-set a lot prior to our meeting, and it was impacting nearly every aspect of his life. I told him he could learn to focus his thinking differently—to steer it in a different direction—and that would help resolve his issues. He was interested to learn. I first took some time to focus on relaxation techniques and then asked whether we should start with a particular area of concern. He suggested basketball. This seemed like a great idea since sports often serve as metaphors for other easily relatable aspects of children's lives.

FAIL AWAY

During his initial introduction to hypnosis, Leo found his relaxing place by visualizing himself playing basketball in an empty gym—a choice that reflected his love for the sport despite his recent performance. Alone on the court in his imagination, he could see the bright fluorescent lights overhead and the empty bleachers, feel the weight and dimpled texture of the ball in his palms, and hear the echo of every bounce and swish as he played. He described the way his feet retraced the same steps over and over as he practiced his layups. In short, he made this unlikely place to find calm sound downright idyllic.

After two weeks of practicing hypnosis at home, however, Leo told me that often he could only see himself stumbling on the court and missing layups. He stopped attempting to relax or self-hypnotize because he was too worried about failing—even in his own imagination.

We had to take a step back, so I suggested he use the imagery of a cloud instead. It has fewer details on which he could get hung up. He could focus on the sensation of it without having to overthink his actions or confront his fear of failure. (Interestingly, when I use this technique with younger children, they often tell me what the cloud tastes like—cotton candy and ice cream are the most frequently reported "flavors.")

After walking Leo through the hypnosis process with our focus on a simple, peaceful cloud, we talked about what would come next. I shared a favorite quote with him, from novelist and playwright William Saroyan: "We get very little wisdom from success."

"What do you think he means?" I asked.

"That we learn from failure?" Leo wondered.

"That's right. And I wonder, how do you think you'd feel if you already knew everything you were going to learn in your life right now, at fourteen?"

"Smart," he said. "And bored, maybe."

"I think so too," I said, "but you're lucky because that's never going to happen. You're always going to be learning. There's always something else we don't know, even when you get as old as I am. People learn by trial and error. We're good at it. I think it's part of what makes us human."

I explained to Leo that I thought he should reframe his recent mistakes on the basketball court and in other areas of his life as learning opportunities rather than failures. If he began to feel anxious, he could take the extra step of mentally noting what he could learn instead of focusing on what he believed he'd done poorly.

"Do you think you could do that?" I asked.

"I'll try."

"Don't try," I said, pausing to let that thought sink in. Leo appeared puzzled.

"Trying leaves room for failure," I clarified. "But when you do something you always succeed, no matter what happens. You either achieve your goal—an obvious success—or fall short of the goal. In the latter case, you learn from your experience and you also come out ahead."

Leo nodded as he considered.

"Some people have a lose-lose attitude," I continued. "They figure they will fail at something, and when they do fail, they feel they've proven their poor worth. If they happen to succeed, they tell themselves that the task was too easy, or that they were just lucky, or that anyone could do it, or that they could have done better—so even their accomplishments don't feel special or satisfying."

"So much comes down to perspective," I added. "You can choose to have a win-win attitude and make that your reality."

Leo thought a bit more. He said, "I'm going to learn from my mistakes."

HOW MUCH IS IN YOUR MIND?

Two weeks later, Leo returned, this time on crutches. He looked miserable. Clearly, he wasn't in a win-win mood.

"What happened?" I asked.

"I wrenched my knee. I'm going to be out of commission for weeks."

"I'm sorry," I said. "But all is not lost. You can still improve even if you can't practice in the gym."

"Why do you think that?"

"Well, what percentage of sports is mental?" I asked.

He thought about it. "I don't know," he said. "Maybe twenty-five percent?"

"Would you believe me if I told you it's a lot more than that?" I asked. "Many athletes have said it's ninety percent. Yogi Berra, of the Yankees, was the most creative about it. He said ninety percent is mental, and the other half is physical."

Leo grinned and said, "I guess math wasn't his thing."

"The upshot is that many athletes are superstars because they know how to think differently. That's what gives them their edge. What do you think of Michael Jordan as a basketball player?"

"Best ever!" he said with great conviction.

"I agree. So, was he the tallest?"

"No."

"Was he the strongest?"

"No."

"The fastest?"

"No."

"Then what made him the greatest? I posit that it's his mind. He knew how to move, how to pass, how to shoot, how to see the whole court and persevere like no other player," I said. "How much of that do you think is mental?"

"Yeah, I see your point."

"Good, because I think practicing in your mind will help you improve even when you are not practicing physically. Want to guess who else used hypnosis to improve his basketball game?"

Leo thought about it for a minute.

"Michael Jordan?"

"The one and only. I think if it's good enough for him, you can certainly give it a shot."

EXERCISE WITHOUT MOVEMENT

Our next step was to lay out a practice schedule that didn't involve playing. We agreed on three mental exercises. The first was the obvious one:

Leo would imagine doing his drills, just as he was accustomed to during practice, for fifteen to twenty minutes each day. As he did this, he'd pay close attention to his form, to how his body was moving and how the ball was responding. He would visualize his teammates and their plays, noting his position on the court relative to the other four players, the basket, and the three-point line. This step would condition his mind to improve those maneuvers.

Second, after each of these visualized practice sessions, Leo would imagine the conversation he'd have with his coach. Because his relationship with the team's current coach had become strained, I suggested he could pick any coach for this exercise—real or imagined, dead or alive.

He considered and then announced he'd choose Phil Jackson—not a surprising selection considering his admiration for Jordan (who played for Phil Jackson as a Chicago Bull) and the Lakers jersey Leo was wearing at a time when Jackson was coaching the Lakers.

I suggested that after each practice he should consult with Coach Jackson, asking him what he might do to improve. Whatever he recommended, Leo should implement in another five to ten minutes of mental practice.

Not surprisingly, Leo questioned this idea. He wondered how he could presume to know what Phil Jackson would have to say about his practice.

Technically, of course, he could not. Neither of us could ask for Jackson's opinion of Leo's virtual basketball practice. Fortunately, this was not the point. This was an intelligent, observant teenager who started playing his sport when he was five years old and had been practicing for a minimum of an hour almost every day for years. He'd been watching games on television all his life. He'd worked under a number of different coaches and watched his peers learn and increase their skills alongside him. None of this made him an expert, but it did suggest he probably knew more about the art of coaching than he'd comfortably give himself credit for. This underestimation of their own knowledge is rife among children and teens who are accustomed to being in deferential roles compared to the adults in their lives.

I asked whether Leo observed errors and missed opportunities when he watched college or pro basketball. He confirmed he did. I asked if he could do the same when he worked out with his teammates or even watched videos of his own play, and he confirmed that as well.

With that in mind, I recommended he have a little faith in his own inner coach—the one that would be taking the form of Phil Jackson.

"You've got this," I told him. "It is well within your skill set to critique your own play, to help Coach Jackson give you advice."

The third exercise I recommended for Leo was imagining himself in a championship game. "Coming in off the bench, you use your relaxation sign to keep calm," I said. "As soon as your feet touch the court, you are on your game, doing exceptionally well. You're throwing great passes and pulling down rebounds and making your shots. You are playing at your best and maybe even winning."

"You can teach your mind to seek that successful, winning feeling as much as possible," I continued.

"Do you think this will work?" he asked.

"The more you practice in your mind, the better you will become. I'm certain."

"How can you be sure?"

"When you apply your mind to any activity that you care about, you improve your mental abilities to perform it. It is a different form of practice than you're used to, but it's practice all the same."

Leo went home in a better mood. He began mental training that evening in conjunction with his hypnosis practice. He stuck to this routine every day for weeks. Each time we spoke, we talked about further aspects of his life in which he could use his new ability to achieve calm and do his best. In some areas, like his diet, we tied things back to basketball—to the importance of fueling his body to stay strong. In others, like his social anxiety, we focused on staying calm and remembering that this is a problem most kids struggle with at some point. When he learned to be mindful that his peers likely also worried they'd say something wrong, he put less pressure on himself to be perfect.

It took six weeks for Leo's knee to improve sufficiently for him to return to the gym without restrictions. He played off the bench for the first week, but when his coach noted his lack of nerves and improved performance, he became a starter again. Over the remaining weeks of the season, he topped every personal record he'd previously set and ultimately helped get his team to the regional championship.

After being out of his routine for a month and a half, Leo surprised everyone, including himself, with his ability to play a high-level game again. During his downtime he had focused on becoming a better player, first in his mind, and then in the physical world.

More critically, during that same time, this patient had made tremendous strides toward managing the anxiety and obsessive-compulsive tendencies that had been dominating so many aspects of his life. He was able to use hypnosis techniques to calm himself at will and to interrupt the cycle of increasing panic he'd been enduring on a daily basis. His family was deeply proud of his commitment and accomplishments— and so was I.

OUT OF THE REALM OF MEDICINE?
Sharing a case like Leo's inevitably brings up one question: Are these kids seeking therapy primarily to gain a competitive edge?

While there are therapists who do focus on these issues as their priority, the answer for my patients in most cases is no. While using hypnosis techniques for sports performance is a common and proven tactic (the list of athletes who've used it includes some of the greatest competitors of all time in their respective sports: Kobe Bryant, Tiger Woods, Shaquille O'Neal, Carli Lloyd, Kerry Walsh Jennings, Mary Lou Retton, Nolan Ryan, and Jack Nicklaus, for starters), the kids who come into my office seeking help aren't there simply to excel. They're there because they have a medical or psychological diagnosis for issues that are interfering with their ability to live productive, fulfilled lives.

For many of these patients, anxiety disorders are the crux of the problem, and when they learn to address those, their satisfaction with their lives improves. For others, however, anxiety and poor performance are components of larger issues that take time to identify, address, and resolve. In my experience, the best way to ensure this happens is to let the patient lead the way. Many children need to build trust before they can delve into the roots of their troubles, and many are themselves not fully aware of all the contributing factors to their issues until they start exploring them in a therapeutic setting. Sometimes we work on enhancement of their sports performance as one of the first tasks because the child is too anxious to immediately address their medical or mental health issues. More often, I discuss hypnosis applications during sports as reinforcement of the self-regulation skills the child has already applied to their symptoms. I treat some patients who need routine follow-up appointments until they feel sufficiently in control of their symptoms and others who resolve one issue and then may return at a later date with another. Once they experience the benefits of hypnosis, most are quite adept at recognizing when they need further help.

USING THE WHITE SPACE

Exploring the usefulness of hypnosis in the context of sports performance paints a vivid picture of its power, but the efficacy of inner resources such as the imagined coach transcends any one aspect of children's lives. As I write this, one of my longtime patients is in her first year of college. Diana's first semester found this brilliant young woman spending several hours each day rewriting her notes by hand after reviewing her original handwritten notes from her lectures because she's found that to be the most effective way to boost her recall. The fact that she was putting in this work shows initiative and commitment, but the routine quickly began monopolizing her days and nights as classes ramped up and the work became more complex.

The fallout was predictable: stress and frustration and a paucity of opportunities to make friends and enjoy her first year of college, all in exchange for excellent grades. When she called to discuss this development, we talked about the truly impressive ability to self-hypnotize she'd developed over our years of collaborating. She had initially come into my practice at the age of thirteen with depression, anxiety, and insomnia so extreme she sometimes didn't sleep for days. She had also exhibited a near phobia of going to school.

She had come a long way from those early days when she moved into a dorm room and embarked on a full academic schedule.

Both Diana and I knew hypnosis was the best tool she had available to address this new concern, so we put our heads together to find a solution she could use to study more efficiently. Time in hypnosis can stretch out or condense at the patient's will, and so I suggested she visualize handwriting her notes on a whiteboard while doing hypnosis rather than actually rewriting them. The method worked! It allowed her to cut her daily study time in half—from nearly eight hours to four. In her newfound free time, she was able to start experiencing other aspects of college life, including joining clubs and making friends.

Using hypnosis enhanced Diana's learning capability by prompting her to fully focus and tap into more of her mental power than handwriting alone allowed.

WHAT YOU CAN DO ON YOUR OWN

From very early on, we raise our children to be students rather than teachers, players rather than coaches. There is nothing wrong with this at all—it's exactly what kids need to tune in and learn. As children age into their teens and beyond, they must learn when and how to pivot by recognizing and trusting their own intellects. Framing this in terms of assuming the role of the coach is an exercise with multiple benefits: tapping into the child's knowledge, raising confidence, and sometimes invoking empathy for the actual coach and the role he or she plays.

Athletes are but one group for whom this mind-set is useful. In academics, the arts, and personal growth, kids can also benefit from stopping to self-evaluate and asking, "What would the coach say?"

Emily's Emergency Response

Positive Intention Is Key

A physician intent on healing is a more effective healer than one intent on making money. An educator intent on teaching is more effective than one intent on maintaining control. Hypnosis is no exception to the truth that intention is a key part of therapy. In fact, because it taps into the realm of psychology, it's a discipline in which the intentions of all parties—patient, parent, and practitioner—can be critical.

Emily arrived in my office when she was sixteen and suffering from unexplained fainting spells. She'd fainted at school multiple times each week for months. She'd had blood work, heart-function tests, and imaging studies to try to determine a medical cause for the spells, which were terrifying to her and her parents, but no medical cause had been found. After reviewing her records and noting the timing of the incidents (always at school, often during specific classes), I suspected that anxiety related to academic stress might be bringing on Emily's fainting.

This kind of response to stress is called a vasovagal syncope, and it boils down to the body overreacting to a trigger. It is fairly common in some circumstances—like at the sight of blood or during an injection—but less so in the day-to-day life of a student. There's no root medical cause, but the psychological trigger nevertheless causes a sudden drop in blood pressure and heart rate that temporarily reduces blood flow to the patient's brain.[1] If the trigger is something rarely encountered—like the sight of a nasty injury—the reaction might not require any intervention. But for a student regularly fainting as a result of feeling overwhelmed by her academics, the condition was disruptive and dangerous. Each time Emily fainted she suffered psychological and social consequences, and each fall put her at risk of injury. This condition needed to be managed one way or another.

I told Emily I could teach her hypnosis and that it would likely help her stop fainting. She was resistant to the idea that psychological stress was causing her problem and told me, simply, "I don't think so."

I answered as I often do with teenage patients who aren't ready to embrace intervention. "When you change your mind," I told her, "you can come back."

I always use *when* rather than *if* to create a framework of expectation. Some kids don't return, but many do. In Emily's case, it took three days—and one more fainting spell in the middle of a school day—before she was ready to use hypnosis.

I asked her why she had come back. She shrugged. "I thought about what you said and realized that I didn't want to keep fainting."

In the end, it took a single session to teach her how to calm her anxiety before it became extreme enough to cause her to lose consciousness. That intervention resolved her issue.

I am certain that if I'd insisted Emily accept help the first time we met, hypnosis would not have worked for her. In that case, she likely would have concluded that hypnosis could not work, and she would have missed out on its benefit. She needed to *want* to do it, as *she* was in control of the hypnosis process. The fact is, it's impossible to separate the power of words from the power of the intention behind them, and this is a matter that patient, practitioner, and parent must recognize.

PATIENT INTENTION

If a patient doesn't want to participate, cooperate, or improve, hypnosis won't work. The vast majority of my patients decide they want to learn and are successful in at least easing their symptoms. Some see marked, life-changing improvements.

I often encounter patients, however, who require some time and reassurance that the decision is up to them before they accept therapy. Many, especially the teenagers, bristle at the idea of needing help or that I might have something to offer them. One recent patient, for example, told his mother he wouldn't get out of the car or enter the office. This was not an auspicious start. Rather than create a standoff situation at a distance, I went to the parking lot and told him he had no obligation to come in—that in fact I'd rather not treat him if he didn't want my help. I explained that I would be unable to help him without his cooperation. I suggested he go home and only come back when he wanted. The spirit of this interaction was neither threatening nor negative; it was a respectful acknowledgment that he was right in believing neither of us should waste our time if he wasn't interested in learning hypnosis. I told him that his mom had scheduled him for sixty minutes of my time, and if he'd like to use it to talk about the problems that had brought him as far as the parking lot, I'd be happy to do so. If not, I'd catch up on some paperwork.

The simple gesture of giving this child the power to make his own decision was enough to pique his interest. He decided to come see the office and maybe help me create a chart for him. As we walked inside together, I asked whether he was a card player, and he said he liked to play rummy. We spent the remainder of his session talking casually about his problems while we played cards. At the start of his next appointment, I found him in the waiting room, ready with a list of questions about hypnosis and why I thought it could help him.

Beyond a simple willingness to participate, kids also frequently need help to adopt a mind-set of self-direction. It's not surprising, given that they are still developing and that many patients are particularly dependent because of physical or psychological health issues. In order to help them be successful in self-hypnosis, I must first emphasize the "self" aspect of the therapy. Once they see that they're doing the work and driving their own results, most kids relish assuming a higher level of command over how they think and feel.

In action, intention translates into success by combining the power of words and images with both the body's and the mind's capabilities. For example, one demonstration I sometimes conduct with patients is having the child stand facing a wall at a distance that allows her to reach out one arm just enough to touch the surface with a fingertip. I then ask her to lift the arm above her head and repeat the word *shorter* several times. When I ask the patient to lower her arm, it typically appears to no longer reach the wall. The patient, knowing better than anyone that she didn't make a conscious effort to cause this outcome, is confused or amused.

When I ask these children what they think happened and whether they believe the arm actually became shorter, most doubt it but aren't sure. When we reframe the exercise, they realize they've subconsciously shifted a shoulder to cause the outcome.

Children learn this is one way hypnosis works. The patient visualizes an image, and then the body translates that image into action in whatever way it can to achieve the intended result. Extending or retracting the shoulder is an easy example—one any child can recognize as logical and physically possible. "What if it is also possible," I ask them, "that other parts and systems of your body are equally willing to accommodate your intentions—to creatively engage in realizing your vision?" In a nutshell, that's exactly what hypnosis helps you do, and I see children utilize that ability every day.

CLINICIAN INTENTION

I believe and teach kids that no matter what happens, things can be better—that they can learn to embrace and work through problems. My most deeply held objective is always to help them achieve more peace and satisfaction in their lives, and doing this involves building trust with each child. Early in my career as a physician, my attitude about healing was quite different—not in my intentions for a good outcome for my patients but in my therapeutic approach. Based on what I'd been taught, back then I was intently focused on the actions *I* could take to help. Over time I've found the best outcomes typically happen when both doctor and patient focus on what *we* can do together. This simple shift has unquestionably helped me become a better physician. It has equally helped many patients maintain and augment their own wellness long after they've finished treatment.

I believe patients recognize this attitude of cooperation in the nature of our relationships, and this becomes an integral part of the healing process. A decade after we first met when he was nine, one young man told me that he remembered most clearly from our first meeting how long I sat silent, waiting for him to formulate an answer to one of my questions. Looking back, he said that was the moment he started trusting that I could help him, because, in his words, "I'd never met a doctor who cared what I thought before."

Ideally, a clinician brings multiple levels of positive intention to each patient and each session. The first among these is the broad intention of achieving beneficial outcomes for the child and being part of evoking those changes. The next is the intention to understand and empower the patient so these changes are self-sustaining. The third is more specific: treatment and session intentions focusing on what the clinician can do this year, this month, this week, and this day to achieve results. This combination of overarching and outcome-driven intentions is a hallmark of effective clinician-patient relationships.

In explaining this concept to children, we often open a dialogue about placebos and their frequently surprising effectiveness. In Emily's case, I asked, "Do you know how when doctors test a new drug, they always check it against a placebo?"

"Sure," she said.

"Do you know why that is?"

"If they give the patient a fake drug that helps, it would show the improvement might be because the patient just believes it works."

"That's right," I affirmed. "And did you know that in studies of new drugs, the doctor also does not know whether his patient is being given a drug or a placebo?"

"Really?"

"Yes," I explained. "We've learned that if the doctor knows a patient is being given a real drug or a placebo, he can convey this knowledge to the patient nonverbally, which can affect how the patient responds. Now you can better understand how a doctor's beliefs and intentions can make a big difference."

"I get it," she said.

"It becomes even weirder," I added. "Did you know that in some studies we see placebos being effective even *after* patients are told the drug is fake?"

"That's hard to believe," she said.

"It is," I said. "I think it works because the patients are told that placebos have helped other patients, and this gives them the idea that they can be helped as well. I think what this also gives us is a little insight into how much power we really have within us to heal when we believe we can heal."

To emphasize this point, I sometimes ask patients (those without food allergies) if they like chocolate. When I asked Emily, she immediately nodded.

I reached to the container on my desk that I keep stocked with Hershey Kisses. "I am going to give you a chocolate kiss," I said as I lifted one from the dish. "But first I'm going to bless it with my intention to help you. Many of my patients have felt better after eating blessed chocolate."

She waited expectantly.

Focusing my gaze on the chocolate, I said, "Emily, I wish you happiness, a good school year, good health, and feelings of well-being and peace."

Then I held out my hand, said, "Here you go," and handed over the chocolate.

"Do I eat it now?" she asked.

"Of course. How else will the intention work?"

PARENT INTENTION

Treating pediatric patients requires a partnership with their parents. For young children, parents often need to help guide their hypnosis. For older kids, parents should usually stay out of the way. Even when adolescents want their parents to help, I encourage patients to use hypnosis on their own as a way of learning how to manage independently. This recommendation implies a belief that the adolescent is capable of independent success, an especially important message when dealing with kids affected by serious and chronic illnesses that necessitate a lot of parent involvement. When we're not sure how involved the parent should be, the best course of action is the most obvious one: ask the *patient*.

Unfortunately, sometimes parental intentions get in the way of a child's healing, particularly when their intentions are more about their own issues than those of the child. An obvious case of this in my own practice occurred with a thirteen-year-old boy who complained of chronic headaches, chest pain, and stomachaches. He had been evaluated at four major medical centers before I met him, and no medical cause could be identified. I recognized his symptoms as ones that frequently arise as a result of stress—and that typically improve with hypnosis. I explained this to both the patient and his parents.

"I'd like to teach you hypnosis and see how you improve," I suggested in our appointment, and then I turned to his parents to add, "If he improves, that would be great. And if he doesn't, we can proceed with a further medical evaluation."

I could see that the patient was interested, listening closely, and nodding. However, his parents were not.

"We're both college professors, and we understand the mind-body connection," his mother explained. "But we don't think this applies to our child."

I wondered for a long time why these parents were uninterested in having their son learn how to help himself. One possibility was that they'd be embarrassed over having taken him to so many doctors if he improved easily. Another is that they believed there was a specific underlying condition for his symptoms and were seeking not exploration but confirmation. A very discouraging possibility is that they subconsciously wanted him to continue to have symptoms. This is a rare but established circumstance, wherein something about a child's illness helps maintain the status quo in a family's dynamics.

Whatever mystery lay behind the intentions of this particular patient's parents, it was not serving his needs in a productive way. With or without hypnosis, this child needed help, and after the extensive explorations that had already been done, it was unlikely he would get it if his parents continued to take the attitude that they knew how to best evaluate and address the problem (though they clearly did not).

Fortunately, most parents approach their children's health issues with the best intentions. Moms and dads simply and sincerely want their children to be happy, healthy, and successful—and those intentions have power in their own right. They drive the search for help, they justify the sacrifices families make to ensure their kids get care, and they enable the nurturing and support that help kids heal and mature. If I could add one dimension to parent intention, I'd advise remembering that in order to have long-term well-being, children must also achieve some level of independence. Parents who make that independence part of their intention for their children tend to be more patient, more supportive, and less commanding of treatment scenarios than those who strive to resolve all problems on their children's behalf.

As parents, we constantly influence our children—what they do, how they feel, how they perceive their own realities. Any parenting effort can benefit from moms and dads being cognizant of this fact and choosing to wield that influence with positive intention.

UNEXPECTED OUTCOMES OF INTENTION

Sometimes the intentions of patient, clinician, and parent come together in unexpected ways. One of my longest-treated and beloved patients was a teenager named Patricia who suffered from anorexia. As with many patients who struggle with this disorder, her eating choices related more to her wish to remain in control of herself than a wish to be thin. Successfully restricting her diet demonstrated this control of her life on the most micro level. Ironically and sadly, in many ways it also prevented her from having control and achieving success in the larger sense of taking steps toward being a fully functioning and self-supporting adult. Patricia was sure that she would fail in the "real world" and clung to this notion even though she was bright, capable, and wise in many ways. By maintaining her anorexia, Patricia ensured that she would be unable to move forward into the "real world" in which her worst fear of failure might be confirmed.

Our early appointments focused on dealing with her anxiety (the reason she was referred for treatment), but this issue was inextricably tied up with her eating disorder. With guidance and practice, Patricia was able to successfully learn hypnosis and use it to eat more healthfully. Over time she gained weight, much to her family's relief, but this was the point at which her intentions and those of her therapy diverged. Patricia's fear of failing to maintain the particular type of self-control she'd established with her anorexia was greater than her fear of poor health. She welcomed my help in managing her anxiety, but she took treatment that involved her diet off the table.

Honoring her decision, as an alternative to hypnosis, I took two rather unusual steps intent on supporting her health. First, I hired her to edit a book project. She was extremely smart and capable, and I hoped the work might build her confidence and sense of self-control outside the realm of diet. She meticulously reviewed my pages for grammatical and syntax errors and made corrections in tidy, miniscule print. We were both proud of her work.

Second, with Patricia's permission, I began scheduling our sessions at lunchtime. Even though she refused any treatment specifically related to her eating, she embraced this new routine. For two years, Patricia, her mother, and I ate lunch together every weekday in front of the aquarium at the children's hospital. Patricia liked looking at the fish, and she identified especially closely with one large orange parrot fish who liked to swim alone, sometimes ascribing feelings to it that I suspect reflected her own. Each day she ate this small meal, readily admitting it was sometimes her only meal of the day.

Those were the last two years of her life. Patricia and I and her family knew all along that her anorexia was killing her, but she could not muster the intention to manage it. To this day, the story of this bright, intelligent, tormented young woman serves as a tragic and powerful reminder about the role of intention in any kind of therapy.

WHAT YOU CAN DO ON YOUR OWN

Years ago I was on a plane when another passenger experienced a medical emergency. In that moment of crisis, the crew made an announcement asking if there was a doctor on board. I quickly set about assessing the fifty-five-year-old man having chest pains and started an IV. Beyond that, I had precious few diagnostic or treatment tools available. I felt even more at a loss as a pediatrician dealing with a serious problem in an adult patient. But I realized that I could offer a supportive, knowledgeable presence and my good intentions for this man's health. Somewhat to my surprise, it became obvious this was valuable in its own right. The man, his spouse, and the surrounding passengers stayed calm. Help was arranged to be waiting at the landing gate. The patient's breathing steadied, and his blood pressure dropped into normal range.

In many ways, parents function every day in the same role I served on that plane. You can't avert every emergency, and you can't always fix things that go wrong, but you can help contextualize the events in your child's life. When bad things happen, you can provide calm, reassuring, competent support. When everyday things happen, you can focus your highest intentions on helping your child develop resilience and self-confidence. When good things happen, you can gently create a context of gratitude. Your intentions for your children are deeper and more complex than simply wishing for their well-being. There are countless ways you can bring these into everyday parenting to help them mature and thrive.

III

THE POWER OF
THE SUBCONSCIOUS

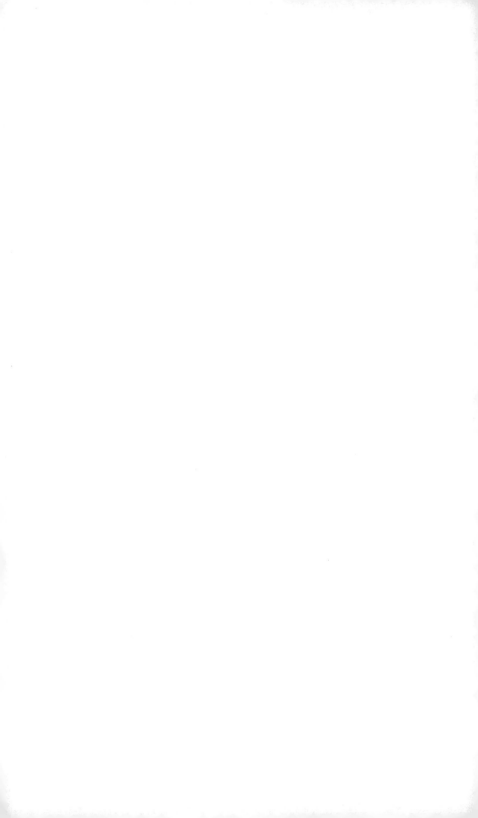

11

The Tip of the Iceberg

Understanding the Role of the Subconscious

In two decades of exploring hypnosis, my glimpses inside the workings of the subconscious have been a fascinating and educational journey unto themselves. Even after all this time, I have a lot to learn—but I also have much to share. Most important, I've found that the subconscious can be a patient's most valuable tool and greatest ally in effective hypnosis therapy.

An oft-repeated analogy uses the metaphor of an iceberg to describe the levels of consciousness of the mind, suggesting that perhaps only 10 percent of its function falls within the realm of the conscious. The other 90 percent is beneath the surface. Much of what we do and perceive occurs courtesy of this vast, often unacknowledged part of our minds. Despite its critical role in almost everything we do—from breathing to remembering to processing emotions—the subconscious is poorly understood. Even the foremost experts in neuroscience, medicine, and psychiatry don't entirely agree about its role and accessibility. To date, contributing to this issue is the fact that the subconscious can't be isolated by any scan or lab workup. It can't be pinned to a single anatomical location or combination of chemical components. The complexity of the subconscious challenges us all and repels the impatient and those who are bound only to absolutes.

I knew very little about the subconscious before incorporating hypnosis into my medical practice. Since doing so, however, I've found it a fascinating, valuable, and surprisingly accessible ally in treating my patients. Figuring out what works, what doesn't, and what is possible is something I've been working on for twenty years—and something I plan to continue studying for the rest of my life.

So how do we define such a complex entity? I tell my patients the subconscious represents the part of their minds of which they are not aware. Everything that goes on outside what they are consciously thinking, feeling, and doing is in its realm. Its functions include the mechanical—keeping bodily functions like breathing and swallowing going—but also the intellectual, emotional, and spiritual. I tell the children and teens I treat that when they stop consciously thinking about something, the subconscious likely keeps turning it over. It is the proverbial "back burner"; it is memory; it is conscience. I suggest that often the subconscious harbors knowledge and wisdom of which they are not yet aware. For young children, I sometimes call it their inner advisor, which is easier for them to both pronounce and understand.

Some clinicians characterize the subconscious and the unconscious as two separate things, with the subconscious working on processes of which we are not aware at any given moment and the unconscious running those that are automatic (bodily functions like circulation and digestion).[1] Since there is no clear line of demarcation, and because this is already a big concept to ask children to grasp, I consider the unconscious part of the subconscious—an entity that commands every internal process of which we are unaware.

I have been asked how I know the subconscious exists and is communicating with me or with the child. One way a clinician can recognize this is when the subconscious possesses and sometimes shares information of which the conscious child appears unaware. Another is in distinctive characteristics (detailed later in this chapter) that it tends to display—characteristics that are often markedly different from the personality of the child. More important from a clinical perspective, as long as the child improves, it doesn't really matter how we label or what we believe about this construct.

Hypnosis is a most efficient and effective way to gain access to the subconscious. There are few clinicians who use hypnosis extensively in their practices, and even fewer who choose to interact with the subconscious directly, but I dove into this realm because of my unconventional introduction to the world of hypnosis and my tendency to follow my patients' lead. As with so many of my experiences in the field, my first encounter with the subconscious came within the framework of my interactions with Paul.

CAN WE TALK?

Once Paul had mastered the art of using self-hypnosis to relax and manage pain, we both felt as though we'd only just begun to scratch the surface of his capabilities. My readings about hypnosis taught me about the possibility of interacting with the subconscious, and Paul was eager to allow his subconscious to communicate with me. I hoped that by learning to interact with his subconscious, I would find an additional angle from which to help Paul overcome some of his well-founded fear of the constant potential for severe allergy complications.

I'd read about the concept of ideomotor signaling, in which ideas are expressed through the movement of muscles. Its documentation goes back to the 1850s and describes the way the subconscious can act and communicate independently of the conscious.[2] Nonverbal interactions often represent ideomotor subconscious interactions. For example, someone might appear sad without even realizing it, while stating that she feels happy. A frown or teary eyes in this case represent ideomotor expressions.

I taught Paul how to allow his subconscious to communicate directly with me in answering simple questions. I asked him to rest his hand on the table next to us and instructed him to leave his hand alone and not to move it on purpose. He learned how his subconscious could signal through his fingers. *Yes* was signaled by raising his pointer finger, while

No, I don't know, and *I don't want to say* were signaled by raising other fingers.

Paul then went to his lake in hypnosis and allowed me to hold as much of a dialogue as was possible with his subconscious limited to those four responses. We started with simple questions, both of us curious as we tested the waters.

"Are you Paul's subconscious?"

Paul's left index finger rose. *Yes.*

I was both delighted and a bit skeptical. "Are you doing this on purpose?" I asked Paul, looking into his eyes.

"No," he reassured me with a surprised expression. "This is happening on its own."

When I recount this experience, this moment often raises the question of how I could carry on a conversation with a patient while he was in hypnosis. The idea that hypnosis is necessarily a passive state is a false one. There are many examples of active hypnosis: athletes who use hypnosis during games, people who drive while in highway hypnosis, and people like Paul who talk during hypnosis. Because of this, I usually ask children to describe their experiences while they are doing hypnosis so that I have a better sense of what is going on in their minds and can guide them and ensure they're comfortable with what's happening during their sessions.

Further, people who become adept at hypnosis are able to easily move in and out of the hypnotic state. When I looked into Paul's eyes and asked him whether he was moving his fingers on purpose, he appeared to come out of his hypnotic state. The clue that he was not in hypnosis at that moment was his surprised expression, as the subconscious rarely displays any emotion in its responses. With that in mind, I turned my attention back to Paul's subconscious.

"Are you willing to help Paul?" I asked, looking at his hand, which was a way of inviting him to reenter hypnosis.

Yes.

"Do you know things that Paul does not know?"

Yes.

There were so many questions I wanted to ask, but it was immediately obvious that this system of communication was going to significantly limit the process. It seemed to me that sticking to yes/no questions would only allow us to scratch the surface of what Paul's subconscious might have to tell us.

The obvious resulting question was "Why can't I just ask the subconscious to talk?"

And so I asked Paul's subconscious whether it would be willing to talk to me verbally.

He raised his left index finger.

Yes.

Of course, the most important permission was still pending. When he was out of hypnosis, Paul and I talked about whether he'd like to let his subconscious speak instead of being limited to the hand signals. Both of us shared an intense curiosity about where this process might lead us, and he immediately agreed and suggested we start at his next appointment.

I eagerly looked forward to more extensive interactions with Paul's subconscious. I wondered what knowledge it might hold. I wondered if it would contain the id and superego, as described by Sigmund Freud, or if it had access to other planes of thought, such as those achievable through prayer. As a doctor, I knew I sometimes saw the subconscious in action. A patient might forget to keep an uncomfortable or inconvenient appointment and then say, "I don't know why I forgot," even though it was pretty clear that on a subconscious level he might not have wanted to keep the appointment. Or patients might talk about dreams that were bothering them. However, observing the work of the subconscious indirectly inevitably involves a lot of interpretation, which can easily be fraught with errors caused by the bias of the interpreter. This would be an opportunity to go to the source, to learn what Paul's subconscious had to say without filters or obstructions. Like most of my patients with chronic and severe health problems, Paul carried a lot of emotional baggage from the experiences of his past. I hoped this interaction might help ease the burden of some of it.

When we met again, I told Paul, "Go ahead to your lake, and let me know when you're there."

Paul took a long slow breath and closed his eyes. In a few seconds, he said, "I see the lake."

In the spirit of our mutual exploration, I had prepared a list of questions, many of them about the purpose and nature of life, and we had agreed I would ask Paul the same questions both in and out of hypnosis to see whether his answers differed. I felt that Paul's self-confidence would improve as he participated in learning about his mind, and I hoped that confidence would serve him well in confronting future life challenges. We also agreed to tape-record the session so I could review what I heard later and also so Paul could hear it if he desired. He wasn't sure whether he would want to listen to the tape, but he liked the idea of having that choice.

What followed was remarkable. When I asked Paul's subconscious questions, he gave me elaborate, articulate answers without hesitation in a low, muffled voice. These were answers he clearly had thought about long before I interviewed him, and they seemed to indicate wisdom beyond his years.

When he came out of hypnosis and looked me in the eyes again, Paul said he didn't recall our conversation. Next I asked him the same questions I'd asked his subconscious in the same order. The difference was startling. Paul hemmed and hawed a lot before answering, and when he did, he gave much shorter answers. Many of his answers were superficial and entirely typical of a teenage boy.

For example, when I asked his subconscious to define love, without hesitation it said, "Love is a special bond that you build with usually one person. I think it's only meant to be built with one. Love is a one-time deal . . . It's an experience that you share with someone, who you care about, who you would do anything for. Go to war for. Die for them. Cry for them. Love is an unchaining of the soul."

This was a profoundly thoughtful answer for an eighteen-year-old, even one who'd experienced the kinds of hardships that tend to deepen perspective.

When I asked, "Where does love come from?" Paul's subconscious said, "It comes from your soul, from your subconscious. From people who surround you. Dead or alive. And from God."

When Paul was out of hypnosis, I asked his conscious self to define love. After giggling for a bit, he said, "Love is . . . I'd have to say . . . See, I don't know, because I've never been in love. I think . . . You know . . . Someone who has been in love can give a better definition . . . My definition is two people who care very deeply for each other."

This, of course, was the kind of answer I'd have expected from someone his age—but it bore almost no resemblance to the answer his subconscious had given. I marveled at how this run-through of my questions almost seemed to be with a different person.

I was impressed that Paul's subconscious answers reflected a more mature view of the world than his conscious ones. I wondered why and how the mind is organized to allow for such a difference.

MANY WAYS TO COMMUNICATE

My work with Paul and his subconscious continued for a year. During that time his subconscious guided and partnered with me in helping him make peace with the things that were most bothering him: his sense of being different from his peers (always a hardship for a teenager) and his fear of becoming ill or even dying from another allergic reaction.

Paul grew and matured tremendously over that year, and through his use of hypnosis he became able to exercise control over aspects of his life that he had felt were spinning out of control when we met. He was able to manage his anxiety, change his perception of pain, and retreat to his quiet lake at will when he was feeling fearful.

The experience opened my eyes to therapeutic possibilities I had not previously imagined possible, and in my role as a pediatrician I began offering hypnosis therapy to patients for a wide range of physical and psychological concerns. Time and again, hypnosis therapy helped where nothing else had made a dent. In patient after patient, hypnosis became a tool of empowerment—giving boys and girls the ability to control what they perceived and how they reacted.

About a fifth of my pediatric patients could not or did not want to allow their subconscious to interact directly with me, and that was fine. Some chose to stick to ideomotor signaling, which turned out to be the easiest way for the subconscious to express itself for most of my patients. Some wanted to speak, and others wanted to write. In time, I had so many writers and was spending so much time trying to decipher their handwriting that I took what I thought was the next logical step— I began asking whether the subconscious would like to type. I rigged up a single computer and monitor with two keyboards, which allowed me to type questions and each patient's subconscious to type answers in response.[3]

When I first started talking, writing, and typing with the subconscious, I was surprised that patients typically did not recall the interactions. Even more surprising was that, before typing, most patients said they wanted to see what they were going to type, but after typing a majority did not want to know what I had discussed with their subconscious. In time I learned that the reason for this decision might be that they were not consciously ready to deal with the topics we covered. With most of these patients, I learned that part of my therapeutic role was preparing them to acknowledge and deal with the issues raised during their sessions.[4]

I believe that my patients chose particular ways for their subconscious to interact with me based on their needs and/or the desire of their subconscious. If patients wanted to be aware of what was said by their subconscious, they would choose to use ideomotor signaling. If they wanted to provide elaborate answers that they would be able to review later, they would choose to write or type. If they wanted to share potentially uncomfortable thoughts without being aware of the process, they might have chosen to allow the subconscious to speak with me.

COMMON CHARACTERISTICS OF THE SUBCONSCIOUS

In my interactions, I've found some characteristics of the subconscious that tend to be consistent, regardless of the age, gender, or history of the patient. Most of my understanding about the subconscious is based on my observations during two decades of regular engagement in thousands of cases. These observations should be considered with the understanding that the subconscious responses can reflect the expectations of both patient and clinician. For example, different patients can have different understandings of what is represented by the subconscious. A clinician who expects the subconscious to yield short answers or believes the subconscious has a limited set of abilities will likely achieve a corresponding response set from the patient. My main bias, based in large part on my experiences with my patients, is that the subconscious possesses knowledge and wisdom of which the patient is unaware. An additional potential bias is that the subconsciouses of patients who do not seek treatment may think very differently from the ones I have encountered. That being said, these are the characteristics I observed:

The subconscious is literal. Early in my exploration of hypnosis, I was mentored by a psychiatrist who used it in her practice. One of the first pieces of advice she offered was to choose my words carefully and keep things simple, because, despite its infinite complexities, the subconscious tends to react highly literally.

In a society where we learn by example at a young age to incorporate irony and double meaning and even passive-aggressive statements into daily conversation, this practice takes some getting used to. The area where I encounter it most often is in the concreteness of patient responses. For example, if I ask the subconscious whether it knows when a patient first developed a particular problem, the subconscious may simply respond "yes." With rare exceptions, the subconscious doesn't elaborate, doesn't ramble, doesn't volunteer information, and doesn't ask questions.

The subconscious is truthful. The subconscious very rarely lies. It may decline to divulge information but almost always appears to be honest in what it does share. I have observed that on a conscious level, patients tend to be concerned with social approval of what they say, but the subconscious does not appear to factor social expectations into responses. One of the reasons hypnosis therapy can be so remarkably effective is because the honest subconscious is deeply knowledgeable about the patient. If the patient is having difficulty processing or expressing an emotion, the subconscious can often pinpoint its origin and articulate it. It can identify thoughts and feelings the patient may be denying or overlooking.

The exception to this expectation is that the subconscious will lie to protect a patient, particularly if it does not want to disclose something that would upset him or her. I avoid prompting such situations by asking preliminary questions about whether it would be OK to ask a particular question rather than forcing a question the subconscious may not be prepared to answer.

Beyond these complex processing issues, the subconscious is also often aware of simpler truths—the forgotten solution to a problem on a test, the code to a combination lock, or even the location of a seemingly lost object.

The subconscious is wise. I treat a lot of teenagers, and a common hallmark of the teen years is the unique juxtaposition between their outward appearances, which are maturing rapidly, and their conscious minds, which often take some time to catch up. The subconscious, however, virtually always seems to behave with the wisdom and maturity of an adult. For example, it often suggests courses of action based on moral rules and long-term expectations rather than convenience or impulse. I've encountered suggestions from the subconscious that I'm certain the child's conscious self has not entertained. The maturity trait is so marked that some years ago I began prompting children to ask their subconscious its age. Surprisingly, in most cases the subconscious claims to be older than the child. Some say they are a few years senior to the child; some indicate ten or twenty years, and some decades. A few claim to be hundreds of years old, and a handful have said that they've existed since the beginning of time. A possible reason for this phenomenon is that it results from my bias and suggestion at the outset of subconscious work that the subconscious might be smarter or wiser than the child.

Regardless of their origin, in my experience these wise older guides within my patients are a blessing to them. In many cases, the subconscious is a steadying force, and the role it plays is like that of the proverbial "angel on the shoulder."

The subconscious looks out for the child. It's been clear in my interactions that in almost all cases, the subconscious prioritizes the child's best interest. The subconscious will refuse to answer questions if it perceives potential harm to the child. It will keep the patient's secrets if telling them could do the patient harm. It will stay true to what is best for the child regardless of the clinician's or society's expectations.

The subconscious can be a source of creativity. On some occasions I've encountered a patient who presents as a typical child or teenager, focused on things like academics and sports and peer groups, whose subconscious writes a poem or draws a picture during a hypnosis session. Most patients do not recognize their writing or artwork after they emerge from a hypnotic state. Often, over the course of therapy with a child, both the patient and I will come to realize the subconscious's creative expression ties into an ongoing issue the patient is working through.

The subconscious is steady. Most of the time, interactions with the subconscious involve nonemotional responses. When a subconscious states it's agitated or anxious, usually it explains that the mood is caused by the patient's anxious feelings rather than its being anxious independently of the patient. For example, if I ask a patient's subconscious, "Does the patient's pain bother you?" the common answer might well be "no." In this way, the subconscious seems to be a step removed from urgent physical and emotional experiences. It is also unpressured by time. It does not rush, and it does not rush the patient if it perceives the patient is not ready to know or confront information or a feeling that might be overwhelming.

I believe that in order to truly appreciate the power of tapping into the subconscious to help heal and empower children, one must see it in action. In the chapters that follow, you'll read some of my patients' stories and see how this powerful and loyal ally helps them work through physical and psychological problems.

WHAT YOU CAN DO ON YOUR OWN

There are times when kids are troubled over a single problem and it's quite possible to help them work through that issue and move on. But it's not uncommon for the obvious problem to be the tip of a different kind of iceberg. Worries have a way of snowballing, each making the previous ones feel heavier. It's a natural reaction to troubled times (whether it's a day or a week or a year) to allow a number of concerns to get emotionally and intellectually jumbled up together until they become an immensely heavy burden. Often, when new patients who are struggling start talking about their troubles, they all come tumbling out. Naming these problems is a useful step in its own right, but the first thing I ask kids *after* they tell me everything that bothers them is whether it would be helpful if they thought about each problem separately. Even when our difficulties and complications are intertwined, we can often find a way to isolate a single issue and deal with it. This positive step—addressing one problem, getting one thing done—gives kids a sense of accomplishment and control. Encouraging children to consider their worries one at a time is an effective problem-solving tactic they can apply to any situation.

Introducing the concept of the subconscious adds another layer to this process by informing (or reminding) children that they possess inner wisdom—that they have reserves of intellect and strength they can draw from to make good decisions for themselves. My appreciation of the wisdom of the subconscious helps me approach children and teens with great respect, which enhances the relationship I have with my patients as a physician and helps promote more effective healing. Parents, too, can remind children they are smarter and stronger than they may think and encourage them to use those assets to help resolve problems one at a time.

A Cough Named Bob

The Subconscious as Cotherapist

Most patients have psychological stressors that contribute before, during, and/or after they experience their symptoms, which are deeply entangled with their personal histories, medical conditions, and habitual triggers. To get to the root of these stressors, the clinician has two choices: (A) send up any number of trial balloons in the form of suggestions—many of which will miss the mark or fail to fly—or (B) allow and encourage the child to voice his or her own reasons so they can be addressed. After twenty years of treating pediatric patients, I've concluded with some certainty that plan B is almost always more effective. There is a unique caveat to this method in hypnosis therapy, though, because in many instances both the patient and the clinician need to have an ally in the process—the child's subconscious mind.

One such case that might well have persisted and eluded treatment without the help of the subconscious was that of a patient named Scott, who was referred to me by another pulmonologist after traditional treatments failed.

As I reviewed the fourteen-year-old's file before his first appointment, I noted that the frequent, severe cough that was his primary symptom had been an on-and-off complaint since he was a toddler. Each time he'd picked up a cold or respiratory virus in the ensuing years, the cough came back. When Scott was twelve, the cough took hold with new strength, and the seemingly uncontrollable coughing fits continued to worsen. They occurred often—as frequently as daily—with some lasting as little as twenty minutes and others hanging on for hours. His symptoms had become so severe that Scott had stopped running track, missed two months of school, and eventually stopped going altogether.

The pulmonologist who referred Scott to me had performed extensive investigations—pulmonary-function testing; tests for acid reflux from the stomach; CAT scans of the sinuses, neck, and chest; an echocardiogram; a study of Scott's sleeping pattern; and even a bronchoscopy. All of the studies had been normal: there was no "smoking gun" that could explain his symptoms. Scott had been prescribed an asthma puffer, asthma pills, nasal allergy spray, liquid cough suppressant, and a pill to control stomach acid—but none of them alleviated his chronic, debilitating cough.

Scott's history rang many bells for me that pointed in the direction of a problem that could be solved with a psychological approach: No one could identify a physical cause of his symptoms, even after many tests, and no medication had helped. His cough was loud and disruptive but never occurred when he was sleeping.

I suspected Scott might be suffering from a habit cough, sometimes called "psychogenic cough" or "cough tic." This disorder, typified by a loud, sometimes honking, chronic, or recurrent cough, can be triggered by a respiratory infection and then continue long after it ceases to be associated with any active disease.[1]

The names this condition goes by might imply the patient is deliberately causing the cough, but that's not the case. Sometimes the cough can be entwined with psychological factors—like a cough that always occurs when a child goes to a place he or she dislikes—but that doesn't mean the child consciously chooses the symptom. In Scott's case, the notes in his chart did not indicate any kind of avoidance.

Sometimes when patients don't appear to have a strong desire to overcome their symptoms, it's a clue that they may be avoiding something else. Scott seemed to want to go to school and run track, but the cough kept him from both. Perhaps most notably, Scott had been dealing with his cough in some form since before he was in preschool. If his symptoms were being caused by a functional disorder, chances are Scott could not remember life without it. I have often lamented that a patient like Scott had not previously met a medical practitioner who could both recognize and treat his functional disorder. His symptoms might have resolved much earlier, even in preschool.

When he arrived in the office, the tall, thin boy gave the room a quick scan and made a beeline for the fish tank, keying in on the bright orange parrot fish. He raised his hand to the glass and then decided not to touch it. Instead, he leaned in, eyes just inches from the tank.

I stepped forward and introduced myself, extending my hand to shake his.

"That's El Magnifico," I told him. "He's the master of the tank. He's almost as old as you."

Scott kept his eyes on the fish but answered. "I didn't realize they got that old."

"Sure. With his cushy life, he might make it to twenty, maybe even older."

As we stood side by side in front of the tank, I told Scott that I was sure El Magnifico knew my face, that he always came to the glass and looked at me when I approached.

Scott turned toward me, brows arched. "You think??"

"Actually," I explained, "there've been studies on this. Researchers have taught triggerfish to squirt water when they see a photograph of a particular person—not just any person. Not only did they do this with accuracy, but they were able to do it even when they were shown a picture of a familiar face in black and white!"

"No kidding?" Scott said, shaking his head and looking at El Magnifico with new respect.

"No kidding," I answered. "I think a lot of creatures are smarter than we give them credit for."

The discussion in my waiting room was an indirect but important part of Scott's therapy. First, we established a cooperative relationship that would serve as a foundation for the positive interactions that would follow. Second, when I talked about the fish being smart, I was providing a metaphorical suggestion to Scott that perhaps people, including him, might be smarter than he realized. I am constantly amazed at the capacity my patients have to be insightful into their own problems and actively engaged in their own therapies when they're empowered to do so.

"Who's with you today?" I asked, nodding to his mother, who stood behind him.

Scott introduced her, and we shook hands.

"Do you want to bring your mother into your appointment?"

Scott paused.

"You can always send her out later, if you like," I added.

"Sounds good," he said. Scott followed me into my office and sat on a chair across from me. His mom sat beside him.

"So, tell me what brings you here," I said to Scott.

His mother began telling me about Scott's medical history. I interrupted as politely as I could manage, thanking her, and asking whether Scott could tell me the rest himself. I explained that there were three reasons for my request. First, I wanted to hear Scott's version of his illness so I could understand what he felt needed to improve. This helps me target my intervention within the patient's frame of reference. Second, if his mother provided his history, Scott might just go along with it, even though her version might not represent his truth. Finally, if his mother provided the history, there would be a subtle implication that Scott could not represent himself well enough to do it. Part of the success of my therapy comes from empowering each child to feel that he or she has the capacity for self-help.

Scott's mother nodded, turned to her son, and waited for him to speak. Scott told me the cough had been part of his life for years, something he always had to deal with. The coughing fits were so extreme, he often had chest pain during and after and a sore throat for hours. He could feel his heart pounding sometimes while he coughed, and that scared him more than anything else.

The soft-spoken boy was very articulate. He described his symptoms, his routine, and his feelings of loss over having to stop running track—a domain in which he excelled.

I asked whether there were any triggers he'd noticed for his coughing events, and Scott said strong odors or the smell of cigarette smoke sometimes started them. He said that he couldn't even go to the mall because the odors of perfume might trigger his cough. Sometimes, though, there was no reason he could detect.

"Do you think you can hypnotize me?" he asked. "Do you think it will help? I've been reading about it, and I think I understand how it works. I used to get bored at school a lot, and sometimes when I'd stare at one spot on the wall, after a while it would start to look different, like I was watching a projector on it or looking through it."

Here he stopped, looking a little shy at confessing to seeing something out of the ordinary, and asked, "Do you know what I mean?"

I nodded. "You're absolutely right. In some ways, the state of hypnosis is simply an extreme level of focus. If you can achieve that on your own, I'm positive you'll be able to benefit from hypnosis therapy here.

"One thing you should know from the start is I will not be hypnotizing you. I'll be teaching you to hypnotize yourself. When you do what I suggest, you can become hypnotized, but only because you choose to do so.

"And one other thing we should talk about," I continued. "The trigger for your cough could be anything—a strong smell, smoke, a cold—and you can learn to control your need to cough when you experience that trigger. I know that sounds unrealistic, because the trigger is something physical, but people have psychological responses to physical triggers all the time. Have you ever felt your heart race when you were afraid of something, maybe a big storm or a scary movie?"

Scott nodded.

"That may be what's happening here. The trigger is the scent, and the psychological response you've been experiencing all your life leads to the symptom of coughing. Your case has one more twist, though, because once you start to cough, doing so causes irritation in your airway—and that irritation is one reason that you *keep* coughing and can't stop.

"So your goal is to stop the cough before it starts. I'd like to teach you to use your mind to shut down that first impulse."

A SUNNY PLACE TO HEAL

Scott chose a peaceful room lined with a wall of tall windows with sunlight streaming through as his relaxing place. He described thick carpet on the floor that felt soft under his bare feet, shelves of books along one wall, and a beanbag chair where he could sit and read and look out at a forest outside. To reach this room in hypnosis, Scott descended a long staircase, breathing slowly and gradually relaxing his body from head to toes. Once there, he said it smelled like pine needles and that there was hot chocolate to drink and warm sugar cookies he could have whenever he wanted. While he was in his relaxing place, I suggested Scott touch his index finger to his thumb, creating a small circle. I told him that from then on, whenever he wanted to relax, he could make that gesture, even when he was not hypnotized, and it would help him feel calm. At the end of this first session, Scott told me the room he visited had seemed vividly real, and when he made the circle with his index finger and thumb, he said he could feel the relaxation he'd experienced in hypnosis.

In order to help Scott learn to control his cough, I suggested he imagine having a coughing fit at school—that he think of the circumstances in which it had been at its worst. He told me he could feel the tickle in his throat, and then he coughed a few times as we were talking, trying to get rid of it. In stressful situations in the past, this is where Scott had lost control. The tickle had become irresistible, and the few small coughs intended to clear it away turned into something bigger and more difficult to manage. He'd cough harder and harder, until the coughing fit was a barking, rasping, full-body experience so severe he couldn't stay in a classroom. His chest would ache, his heart would pound, and he'd feel there was nothing he could do to stop any of it.

We needed to figure out some system to stop that process before it got out of hand. Scott was an eager and creative participant in his therapy, so I asked him what imagery he thought he could use to interrupt the tickle before it turned into a full-blown cough. We talked about the possibility of a numbing liquid, but Scott associated that with a liquid he'd had to drink for one of the tests he'd taken to diagnose his problem—and he didn't want to feel that way again. We considered ice chips, but he didn't think that would work because the trickle of melting ice might cause a tickle rather than alleviate it. We discussed imagining the color of the cough changing from red to orange to yellow to white and neutralizing it, but he wasn't confident in that strategy either.

In the end, it was Scott who came up with the suggestion that would stick. He decided he would imagine himself eating cold grapes and feeling the cool, smooth fruit soothing the tickle in his throat as they passed it.

At our next appointment, Scott reported that he'd had some success with his relaxation techniques and with imagining eating the grapes, but his cough still kept returning. We'd both hoped he'd be able to clear it up completely.

I asked whether Scott would allow me to speak with his subconscious during that day's hypnosis session. Perhaps it would be able to help me understand why the cough was lingering. Scott was keen to cooperate, so I explained how it's possible for a person to act without being consciously aware of it during hypnosis. In this case, Scott could allow his subconscious to answer questions using ideomotor signaling or even by writing answers or speaking with me directly. At the end of the session, I could share what his subconscious told me, or I could keep it to myself if he preferred. It was up to Scott to decide.

Scott wanted to know what his subconscious might say. He liked the idea of letting his subconscious write, and with those ground rules set, I talked him through going back to his relaxing room, while he held a pen in his right hand, poised over a piece of blank paper. Once he achieved a state of hypnosis, I suggested, "Once your subconscious is ready to write, he can write *Hello.*"

A few moments later Scott's hand touched the paper with the pen tip and wrote *Hello.*

"Am I speaking with Scott's subconscious?" I asked.

Yes.

"Will you help me try to cure Scott's cough?"

Yes.

"Do you think Scott will be willing and able to give up his cough?" I asked.

Yes.

"He has been making improvements," I said, "but the cough is still there. Why is it hard for him to let it go?"

At this point, Scott hunched over his paper, writing. I waited until he sat up and laid down his pen.

The cough is bad. But Bob is part of Scott.

I was confused.

"Is Bob the cough?" I asked.

Yes.

"Can you explain how Bob is part of Scott?" I asked. "Is it like an appendix? Because a person can give up an appendix and never miss it."

It is part of Scott, like part of his soul.

"Can Scott function without that part of his soul?" I asked. "I think he might be better off without it."

Again, Scott leaned forward to write. When he set his pen down, he had drawn a circle, like a pie, with a wedge cut out of it. Beside the circle the subconscious had written, *A part of him would be missing.*

I thought for a moment about how the subconscious had explained clearly why it was so difficult for Scott to give up his symptom. I used the subconscious's explanation to help formulate my next suggestion: Once Scott allowed the cough to leave, the pie could fill in, and he would feel better. By continually building off of the ideas provided by Scott's own subconscious, I prompted it to act as his cotherapist and acknowledged its active role in his treatment.

The response was, *That might work.*

As Scott's subconscious seemed tentative, I tried a different tack. "Could you make a deal with Bob that it can stay as long as it doesn't cause Scott to cough? Would that be possible?"

Scott's subconscious wrote, *Yes. That could work.*

With Scott's subconscious's stamp of approval, I felt comfortable moving forward. "Will Scott remember this discussion?" I asked.

Yes.

When Scott came out of hypnosis, I showed him the notes and the diagram. He didn't indicate any knowledge of his cough having a name or any idea why it might be named Bob, but he thought the deal might work.

When Scott's mom came in, he told her in great detail about what had transpired, showing her the pie drawing and talking about his cough named Bob. I could see her skepticism, but it was difficult to argue against the eager hope for a cure she was seeing in her son.

A few days later Scott sent me an email thanking me and describing his interaction with Bob since he'd left the office. "I've been in contact with scented candles and perfume, and Bob only gave a slight notification that he was annoyed," Scott wrote. "I didn't cough. And I didn't need any medicine."

Scott's letter closed with "Bob says bye, hopefully."

When I spoke with Scott's mother, she described how the family had gone to the mall, knowing there would be strong scents that might trigger a coughing fit. It was a test, and he'd remained calm. She noted that every time she looked at him, he was holding his thumb and index finger together, his relaxation sign.

After a week with no coughing fits, Scott returned to school. I continued to see him for another three weeks, and the cough stayed away. At our last appointment, Scott reported how relieved he was to finally be free of it. He said his biggest concern was whether his subconscious had somehow been causing his symptoms for years. He wanted to know why it would do that, and he wondered, if it would do that to him, what else might it do to harm him? Was it evil? Might it try to take him over? What had happened to him, together with the fact that he felt betrayed by a part of himself, was a lot for Scott to process.

I told Scott I'd yet to meet a subconscious that didn't have the best interests of its conscious being as its main focus. Whatever process had led to his body hanging on to the habit cough, it likely had more to do with the difficulty of giving up a symptom that had come to feel like a part of Scott's identity than with intent to do him harm.

Five months later, Scott's mother sent me an update. He was going to school every day and making good grades, he was off all his medications, and he was training for a marathon. Bob, if it was still somewhere deep in his subconscious, was dormant, and Scott was getting on with his life.

Scott's family did a beautiful job of supporting him throughout his therapy and the process of gaining control over his triggers. The family plays an important role in this process, and Scott's struck an ideal balance between encouraging him and respecting that he was in charge of helping himself.

Scott's case taught me an important lesson about how a functional symptom can become completely integrated into a patient's identity. I've since encountered other patients who need help letting habitual symptoms go, and I've learned that freeing children from those symptoms often involves not just addressing the problem but also partnering with the subconscious to figure out what adjustments are necessary for each patient to find a new normal. For some, like Scott, the transition may take just a few weeks. For others, it is a process that can take months or years.

WHAT YOU CAN DO ON YOUR OWN

All kinds of psychological reasons—sometimes with physical triggers—can contribute to kids' physical symptoms. For example, if a patient's heart races when they view a scary movie, the physical trigger (viewing the movie) has caused a psychological response (fear) that led to a physical symptom (the racing heart). These things happen all the time in the context of our daily lives, but when they begin to become routinely disruptive, it's time to start working to resolve them.

While there is no substitute for getting professional help, you can make a point of encouraging children to voice the reasons they perceive to be contributing to their symptoms. If your child has frequent headaches or bellyaches, for example, ask whether anything is happening at the beginning of the events or whether anything seems to make them worse. This will cause the child to start thinking about triggers. Initiating this conversation implies not that the symptoms the child experiences are any less real but that maybe there's something they can do, perhaps with your help, to ease them. It's a small but important first step in connecting the dots between the way the child feels and their finding a measure of control to help improve their symptoms that they may not have realized was at their disposal.

13

The Poet and Dave Matthews

Opening Pathways of Creativity

The inability to understand and express pain or discomfort can contribute to physical symptoms and to difficulty moving past them. We often see this in young children who may be unable to distinguish between physical discomfort and emotional distress—leading to things like crying "Ouch!" at even a gentle touch when they're upset or becoming overwhelmed by a small inconvenience when they're physically sick. Of course, this happens to adults too, as almost all of us know someone who gets short-tempered and irritable when they get hungry (also known as being *hangry*). This blurring of the lines is a phenomenon I frequently observe in patients suffering from a wide variety of ailments. Kids require the right words (or some other form of self-expression and communication) to fully process and convey what they feel and need.

Many patients find this missing piece by tapping into their creativity and discovering new ways to express themselves. The subconscious can play a vital role in sparking that creativity. This was the case for one of my patients, a boy who was tormented by persistent abdominal pain. I suspected from the beginning that he had a vivid imagination, as his was one of the most surprising imagined relaxation places I've encountered. Most kids choose a quiet place for this exercise, but Ian opted to imagine descending ten stories in a hotel elevator, arriving at a

Dave Matthews Band concert on the bottom floor. To date, he's my only patient who has chosen to visit a rock concert to relax.[1]

Ian was referred to me not by another physician but by his older brother, Steve, who was about to age out of my care as a pulmonary patient. Steve suffered from asthma, and as a teen he'd dangerously misused his medications. I'd worked with him to change this behavior, and he in turn had joined my asthma education group and helped instruct other teenagers on the importance of managing their meds. He'd done such a great job, I asked if he'd like to be featured during the hospital's Children's Miracle Network broadcast, and he'd been honored to be included. At the age of twenty, he came for a final visit and told me about his brother, whose severe abdominal symptoms—something he'd lived with most of his life—were keeping him from going to school on a normal schedule.

Ian, a creative, intelligent sixteen-year-old, had endured every physical test imaginable to diagnose his problem, and even though doctors believed they had it pinpointed multiple times, the treatments for those diagnoses brought no results. Ian had undertaken a number of different restrictive diets that had no impact on his pain. He'd been evaluated by a psychiatrist and put on an antidepressant, but that didn't help either. Despite every intervention, this teen woke up most mornings with stomach cramps that would worsen and eventually lead to diarrhea and pain so intense he couldn't function at school.

The first thing I told Ian when we met was that I'd do what I could to help him identify the root of his problem. That said, because pain was at the center of his torment, I was confident I could help him feel better regardless of whether we ascertained its specific physical origin. He wanted to know why I was so sure, and I explained that hypnosis can usually modify perception of pain regardless of its cause or, at the very least, improve patients' ability to cope with their discomfort.

I often tell my patients they shouldn't use hypnosis to ignore new or different pain in case it might have an urgent medical origin. For a patient like Ian, who had lived with cramps and bellyaches that did not improve for years despite medical evaluations and therapies, it was safe to assume being able to compartmentalize his pain would improve his daily life.

IF YOU CAN START IT, YOU CAN END IT . . .

After Ian had learned the basics of self-hypnosis, I helped him learn techniques to reduce his perception of pain. The first of these involved associating the warmth of light with pain relief.

"Imagine a bright light above your head," I suggested. "I'm not sure what color the light is—it might be white, yellow, or red or any other color you imagine. This is a healing light. As it passes through your body, it will heal every nerve, every fiber, every muscle, and every cell in your body."

Then I suggested that the light enter Ian's head and work its way through his body, especially concentrating on his abdomen.

When he completed this hypnosis experience, Ian reported that the light felt warm and pleasant. He said he was very relaxed and that the experience felt real to him. His pain had subsided, and he was comfortable.

Because this was a problem that had plagued Ian for more than a decade, I suspected he would require more than one tool to manage it. With this in mind, we talked about how a person who can cause something to start can also cause it to stop. I asked Ian to re-create his abdominal pain with the use of hypnosis, which he did, describing it as a seven on a scale of zero to ten. Then I suggested he turn that pain off, and he was able to do so immediately. Thus he demonstrated to me, but more important to himself, that he could diminish his pain at will.

The next week, Ian reported that he had been pain-free for five days—a huge improvement over the handful of pain-free days a month he'd been experiencing before learning hypnosis.

These first steps toward healing piqued Ian's interest in how hypnosis works and what else he could accomplish. Because he was eager to explore it further and was still having some painful days, I asked if he would like to let his subconscious converse with me. He wanted to try this and quickly learned to allow his subconscious to type.

SOMETHING TO SAY

I was surprised to find that the subconscious wasn't necessarily interested in participating in a problem-solving exercise in the form I'd been using with many of my patients. This time the child's subconscious had something to express, something that would become a talking point for conversations to follow with Ian.

It came in the form of a poem:

This feeling I get sometimes
Like an internal blast
Ready to explode
How long will it last

Waiting, feeling, not knowing what to expect
When will the suffering end
No medicine to heal me
How far will I bend?

Intense at times
I struggle to see
What's always lurking
Inside of me.

Thirteen years of chronic, bottled-up pain had left a mark. When I asked whether Ian's subconscious had anything to say about hypnosis, that answer also came in the form of a poem:

All these senses I feel deep inside
Deafening silence to my ears
A cold breeze on my skin
Give me goosebumps as I stare into space

The feel of the cloud is warm and soft
like a comforter by a fire . . .

All this I feel in a moment's time
Every second may differ in various ways
but I try to remember the good feelings
of being safe and calm and relaxed . . .

There was a lot to be hopeful about in that assessment, and I was excited to hear what Ian would have to say about it and about the relationship between the two poems.

When Ian finished hypnosis that day, he denied having knowledge of either of them. He was surprised to find out that his subconscious had the ability to compose complete creations and that not all of these had yet been revealed to him. Ian wondered whether he could use his subconscious abilities to help write music for his band. Further, he continued to write poetry during subsequent appointments with me. Expressing himself in verse helped him deal with his feelings of anger and regret over having lived with pain for such a long time.

A few months after our first appointment, I met with Ian and his mother and discharged him from my care. He had been pain-free for weeks and was back to a regular school-day routine.

His mom hugged me as they left, saying simply, "Thank you so much."

"You know," I mused, "Ian's improvement has been so dramatic I'd like to nominate him as a candidate for this year's Children's Miracle Network broadcast."

His mother laughed. "So then I'll have two miracle children."

That's right, I thought—one helped with modern medications and one helped with hypnosis. It was clear to me in looking at these two brothers that neither therapy was less essential than the other.

EXPLORING CREATIVITY THROUGH HYPNOSIS

For as long as human beings have been writing and creating music and art, we've been trying to find ways to get in touch with the parts of ourselves that inspire and inform. We instinctively know they are crucial to both experiencing our *Aha!* moments and recording them through some form of satisfying self-expression. In the working world, we call these valuable stretches, when we become truly immersed and productive, *flow*. During these moments, we feel disconnected from time and distractions and entirely focused on the task at hand. Not having to agonize over the details, because we find them at our fingertips, we are ready to write, paint, sing, or build. These are times when productivity comes quickly and easily. Artists have described it as channeling a source, being a conduit for ideas, or having the right expression pour out of them.

The state of flow and the relaxed focus that's uniquely achievable in hypnosis have much in common. In fact, it's arguable that flow *is* a form of hypnosis, similar to the forms I point out to my pediatric patients when we first meet. If they have become lost in a book or a daydream, or if they've walked or biked or driven to a destination as if on autopilot, they've already had hypnotic experiences.

Knowing these concepts are closely related, there is an entire contingent of hypnosis practitioners who specialize in helping people access and harness their creative talents by learning to relax, block out distraction and doubt, and focus on a single objective or challenge.[2]

Ian's case helps explain where much of that expressive and fulfilling creativity may originate. Its source often may be rooted in the subconscious, the part of ourselves that regulates, processes, and controls so much of who we are and what we do—without us having to think about it. That this entity—this biggest piece of the iceberg of the human mind's capability—would help us process ideas and art and conflict makes perfect sense. It already quietly does the work of keeping us functioning, keeping track of details of our lives that don't enter our conscious thinking, so that we can, for example, keep driving even while daydreaming or imagine a scene from a book as a full, live performance in our heads.

In my career I've encountered subconscious interactions that involve not just finding the right words to write but also determining musical notes to play (which the patient remembered and recorded after hypnosis) and imagining the colors and lines of a painting the patient was able to re-create on a canvas. In essence, these children and teens demonstrated that the subconscious is capable of thought and creativity of which the patient is not consciously aware.

And yet Ian, like many other young people who practice hypnosis, took a cue from his subconscious and expanded his own practice of writing poetry. In some way, he took ownership of the creation of his subconscious mind, making the effort to understand it, recognize himself in it, and expand on it with further works. Hypnosis became a tool that allowed him to access this other knowledge base and to begin to think with both parts of his consciousness—both minds—at once.

A CREATIVE TOOL FOR WELLNESS

The ability to tap into the creative powers of the subconscious may seem like a small benefit for children with physical or psychological health issues, but in my experience it's powerful. Creative expression has a number of known health benefits for people of all ages, as well as some that are less understood.[3]

First, creativity is tied to providing a valuable outlet for patients to articulate and express complicated and deeply held feelings. Emotions like Ian's lingering sorrow and regret about the physical ordeal of having suffered stomachaches for so long need to be shared and dealt with, and his poems became the first steps in his doing that.

Second, writing, drawing, sculpting, and some other creative outlets have been documented to help patients with all kinds of physical and psychological ailments take ownership of their hardships.[4] In doing so, they can begin to define how those hardships fit into their life stories. For example, many children come to believe (and I agree) that their suffering has made them more empathic and understanding people. Some believe it has made them more artistic or expressive. Some feel it gives them a unique perspective on the world, thereby helping to make them unique and special.

In addition, writing, composing, or playing music and other forms of creative expression have been associated with better management of chronic pain, boosted immune function, and other seemingly concrete measures of good health.[5]

The exact correlation between creative expression about important and stressful events and improved health is not well understood. This practice, however, like nearly everything in hypnosis therapy, has no downside. Children willing to express themselves about the physical and emotional hardships in their lives in essays, poems, music, paintings, or any other format frequently find help in coping with those troubles. Deliberately asking the subconscious to be involved through this process during hypnosis is a valuable addition to it. Even without any direct interview, though, kids often let glimpses of feelings they haven't yet fully processed through conscious thought rise to the surface and onto the page.

I had a thirteen-year-old patient, Benjamin, who initially came to see me for persistent vertigo. In the process of resolving that issue, he began writing poems, first with his subconscious leading the way during our sessions and eventually on his own, with and without the aid of active hypnosis. As part of our work, I suggested Benjamin start to journal regularly. In the weeks and months that followed, he returned again and again with poems he said just poured from his fingers, ones he didn't have to think about at all. When we asked his subconscious about these free-flowing poems, it explained that they were not *from* the subconscious but had been channeled *through* it. They were, of course, Benjamin's thoughts and words, but they came from a deep part of his psyche with which he might never have found a way to connect without the help of hypnosis.

I was continually surprised by the sophistication of Benjamin's poetry, which illustrated the depth of knowledge and ability that was accessible through his subconscious. Take, for example, the first poem he wrote in his journal:

Who are we
A race of loam set to traipse the trees
Perhaps we need to conquer the seas
And crest the rising foam

Who are we
This race of man with power to change the world
We play at God yet sorely flawed
Our tapestry unfurled

What are we
A race of soul with spirit and mind beyond
Through it all we search for hope
Our passion wild a bucking foal
Wavering through the frond

Why are we
Placed here in this world anew
Yet we search for answers
Never ending never finding what is true
When are we set to end our maddening search for soul
Time is perpetual a flowing trend
Chronology set to roll

How are we
Not destroyed wasted by our will
The winds of man our preening frill
Echoed by the void

Where are we
Existing in endless void
Looking for reference searching forever

Doomed to never see
Isolated with no deference
Never finding me.

Benjamin's work helped him process many of the challenges of growing up, as well as the pressure he felt to perform in school. Along the way, it also made him a beautiful poet, one with a nuanced voice and a masterful command of vocabulary.

The idea of muses and creative inspiration and being a conduit for words or notes or art is nearly as old as human civilization, but it is nonetheless exceptional that many of my patients, like Ian and Benjamin, are able to access this way of expressing themselves fully and eloquently so early in their lives. Each of them has benefited immeasurably from the experience, and each now in part defines himself in terms of this laudable and productive accomplishment.

WHAT YOU CAN DO ON YOUR OWN

Tapping into the subconscious can help patients more readily access their creativity, but the value of creative expression isn't limited to any single corner of medicine, psychology, or parenting. Any child can benefit from working through things in writing, for example. Studies have shown that prompting patients to write down their thoughts about important events in their lives is helpful in improving medical illnesses such as asthma.[6]

Journaling is effective on many levels, especially for kids. It can help them define their own stories and work through complicated feelings—something children with medical and psychological issues have in great supply. As a bonus, it can also improve overall writing and communication skills.

Journaling is a self-directed activity that can't be forced, but you can encourage it by providing a cool diary or notebook to write or draw in, setting aside a quiet time and place for its use, and modeling a little journaling of your own.

Dreams of Wolves, Dying, and a Protective Universe

Using Hypnosis to Understand Dreams

There are many subtle (and not-so-subtle) ways in which a child's subconscious may interface with their conscious thoughts and actions. This happens during everyday activities as well as at times when kids are struggling with physical and psychological challenges. Creative outlets, like the poems Ian relied on to help him make peace with years of living in pain, are one example. Dreams are another. The surreal nature of dreams and their ability to evoke powerful emotions can make kids feel overwhelmed, especially when they're unable to interpret nightmares that haunt their sleep.

Sigmund Freud referred to dreams as "the royal road to the unconscious," and they are an area in which hypnosis can be especially helpful in getting to the core of whatever idea or emotion is at work.[1] I've helped many children work through interpreting and making peace with troubling dreams, sometimes because the nightmare itself causes problems, such as fear of going to sleep, and sometimes because it is the subconscious's way of insisting another emotional issue be dealt with.

EASING THE GRIP OF FEAR

When children are losing sleep and peace of mind to bad dreams, they typically remember just fragments—often the scariest ones. As a clinician, I've learned to encourage and enable them with hypnosis to follow these dreams from beginning to end to find resolution.

This was the method I used to treat Olivia, whom I met beside the fish tank in my office waiting room when she was eight years old. When I stepped up to introduce myself, I was surprised to realize that the fish this child was intently watching was Anthony, the upside-down catfish. Her interest in the creature was not surprising (he's a funny-looking little fellow with spotted coloring and long, dangly whiskers), but his presence near the glass in the middle of the day was not a common sight.

"We usually only see Anthony at night," I said. "There must be a reason that he came out to meet you this early in the day. You must be pretty special!"

The little girl turned her wide brown eyes to me. She gave me a shy smile, and her round cheeks dimpled.

I introduced myself and invited her and her parents into the office. Olivia sat snuggled close to her father, and the family told me she'd been increasingly tormented by a recurrent dream of being chased by wolves. The nightmares had started when Olivia was four, after she'd been chased by a large dog in her neighborhood. At first, her parents thought she'd outgrow her nightmare, but in the ensuing years the dream had gotten worse. Olivia would wake two or three times a week, crying and sometimes screaming in terror, and then run to her parents' room for comfort.

Long-term sleep deprivation can wreak havoc on anyone's physical and psychological health, and in this case it was impacting the entire family.

I told Olivia I'd met many patients with nightmares, and, as with Anthony the fish's appearance in the daytime, there usually was a reason for their dreams. I explained that I have taught my patients that by using hypnosis to experience their scary dreams all the way to the end, they'll be able to stop having them.

"Why?" she asked—an excellent question.

I explained that while the answer might differ depending on the person and the dream, there was a good chance her mind was trying to work through something, and if she experienced the whole dream, she'd be able to understand its meaning. Once the meaning was understood, there would be no need for the dream to recur. There was little reason to delve deeply into the concept of the subconscious with a child under these circumstances, but my expectation was that Olivia's subconscious had something to express that had been stymied for a long time—so long that perhaps at this point the dream was more a habit than an expression of fear of dogs.

As I became more experienced at hypnosis, I learned that it often has the ability to reveal whether a psychological dilemma is the *cause* of a problem or a child's *solution* to one—and in either case hypnosis can help bring the situation to resolution.

Olivia readily agreed to go into hypnosis and easily imagined her dream. I asked her to describe it to me as it happened.

"I'm being chased by big grey wolves. They're coming closer and closer," she said.

"Keep going," I said.

"They get closer and closer no matter how fast I run." She gave a deep sigh, more like a weary old woman than an active, imaginative child. She'd been here before. "The wolves are catching up!"

She opened her eyes and looked at me. "I'm scared," she said. "This is when I wake up."

"You're doing a great job," I said. "This is a safe place, and I'm going to stay here with you. I would like you to keep going so you can find out what happens in the dream *after* you wake up."

Olivia nodded and closed her eyes again. "The wolves are getting so close. I'm afraid they're going to eat me. But now I fall into a hole."

"Go on," I said, pleased Olivia was able to get away from the wolves and move past the point when she usually awoke.

My sense of encouragement ended at her next update.

"I fall down the hole and I land in hell. The devil starts chasing me. He's big and hairy and *so mad*. He's getting closer!"

I wondered why this eight-year-old was imagining herself in hell, but I trusted my history with this technique and encouraged her to keep going.

"He's reaching out his big, clawed hand. He's going to catch me!" she said, her voice shaking.

I reminded Olivia she was in a safe place, that this was just a dream, and asked her to keep going.

"He catches me. And he squeezes my neck. And he kills me."

This was obviously not the ending I'd hoped for. I marveled at all the fear this child had bottled up. I said, "Go on," again, wondering (and worrying a little) where the dream could go from there.

"The devil takes me up to the surface of the world," she said. "He tars and feathers me. Birds are swooping down, and he's fighting them off so they won't take me."

At this point I was thinking that perhaps my dream resolution approach was not going to work and also considering where this cherubic eight-year-old had encountered and internalized the idea of being tarred and feathered. I hoped there was a positive, or at least useful, plot twist coming as I encouraged her to press on, asking, "What happens now?"

There was silence for a minute as Olivia played out the end of the dream, something she'd never before seen. With her eyes still closed, she grinned, her cheeks dimpling again, and my hopes rose.

"Oh!" she shouted. "It's angels! Angels come!" She sounded so surprised, practically singing out the words. "Angels come and chase away the devil. And they bring me back to life."

I began to breathe more easily.

Olivia opened her eyes wide, sat up, and looked at me with a confidence I had not yet seen in her. "And *that*," she concluded triumphantly, "is the end. That's the end of my dream!"

"What do you think the dream means?" I asked.

"It means God protects me!" she exclaimed.

"That's right," I concurred. I loved the idea that this child had come to such a hopeful conclusion, but no matter what resolution she'd found to the long-running nightmare, I was confident it would have been the right one for her. Further, I realized how wrong I was to assume that her recent nightmares reflected her fear of animals. Instead, while the content of the nightmares—being chased by wolves—remained the same over the years, the reason for them appeared to have changed at some point to reflect an older child's struggle with existential questions.

I never saw Olivia again after that appointment. Her dad reported that the nightmare no longer recurred. Seeing it through had purged it from her routine. On the rare occasion the topic came up, she would simply remind her parents that "her" angels rescue her at the end.

A SHIFT IN PERSPECTIVE

Olivia's fears may have been blown out of proportion relative to their origin and easily resolved by helping her regain a sense of self-direction, but many patients deal with fears and anxieties that have no simple solutions. This is especially true for those with severe and chronic health conditions. One of these patients, a young man named Jared, left an indelible mark on my life.

As an aspiring physician in med school, I was taught to engage patients with "detached concern." In theory, this level of connection gives patients the empathy they need while insulating doctors from the potentially overwhelming emotions of caring deeply. It is supposed to protect against biased treatment decisions as well. This approach has never worked for me (or for many other physicians), as I haven't been willing or able to separate medical care and emotional care. Instead, over the years I've developed close relationships with many patients and their families, but I've worked on being able to attach and detach as needed. If a patient needs me, I want to be there fully. If they do not, I've learned to take a step back.

My patient Jared, who lived with cystic fibrosis, invited me wholeheartedly into his life, and I accepted. In addition to being his pulmonologist, I considered myself his friend and at times strove to be his mentor. I knew his family, and he knew mine. I met his girlfriend, attended his graduation, and wrote him recommendation letters for college. Jared, perhaps in some small part because of our trusting relationship, faithfully adhered to the extensive and uncomfortable regimen of daily treatments that helped manage his breathing. He learned to perform self-hypnosis and used his skills to help himself achieve calm and tolerate the discomfort of his treatments. Despite the severity of his disease, he was leading a full life.

When Jared was twenty, a ruptured blood vessel in his lung nearly brought his life to a sudden and tragic end. During that terrible event, Jared stated he did not want to have a breathing tube inserted into his windpipe, because the severity of his lung disease would likely cause him to die even while on a ventilator. He said that he did not want to suffer in this way. This was a young man who had grown up in the uniquely frightening position of knowing his chronic condition would be fatal, not in some far-distant future but while he was still young.[2] Not long after the trauma of that incident, though, he began having recurrent fears and nightmares about coughing up blood. The feelings were so intense that they prevented him from falling asleep easily at night, and they kept him on the sidelines of his normally physically active life because he was afraid of an injury. He said that even thinking about bleeding caused his chest to tighten and his heart to race.

To help with Jared's anxiety, I suggested during his hypnosis that whenever he felt his heart beat fast, he could imagine it sending waves of relaxation emanating through his body. The image helped him feel calmer, but it did nothing to ease the torment of the nightmares he also was experiencing. He agreed to use hypnosis to allow his subconscious to show him the nightmare.[3] We both hoped this would help him find a way to stop its recurrence.

In the quiet of my office, Jared, who had years of experience with hypnosis, slipped into a hypnotic state with minimal guidance. I instructed him to allow the bothersome recurring dream to start and asked him to raise his hand when he reached the part when he usually woke up.

Jared appeared to focus intently for a few moments and then raised his hand.

I suggested that he put his hand down, as it had remained floating in the air because he was deeply immersed in hypnosis. "Now, continue to dream the dream to find out what happens at the end," I instructed.

Barely a minute later, Jared opened his eyes and gave me a nod.

"What happened?" I asked.

"The dream has two endings," he explained with surprising calm. "In one I lived, and in the other I died."

This was not what I'd expected, and I waited to hear how he interpreted what he'd seen.

"I realized that no matter which ending occurred, I'd be all right," he said. "My suffering wouldn't last a long time."

Though his health challenges persisted and eventually worsened, Jared's nightmares no longer recurred. When we talked about why this was so, it became clear that this brave young man had not been exceptionally afraid of death. He'd lived with the specter of it all his life. His nightmares had instead been the result of his fear of prolonged pain and distress. He took the opportunity of facing the fear in his nightmare to reiterate his wish not to be intubated or kept alive on a ventilator, and he accepted that the closure he'd found in his dream with two endings—the assurance that possible future suffering would be short-lived—would one day come to pass.

SELF-DIRECTED SOLUTIONS

Parents who are aware that dreams are frequently a vehicle for communication from the subconscious can be mindful that a recurrent dream may indicate an unresolved issue that can be dealt with through hypnosis therapy. For some of my patients, like Olivia, this is the end of the problem. For others, like Jared, the dream may offer a way to better cope with deeper and more complex medical and psychological issues.

The evidence for this is in how often recurrent dreams cease after patients witness them to the end and interpret them for themselves. A critical component of this process is the child's interpretation of their own dream. A clinician can ask questions and provide guidance, but the child needs to recognize and accept an interpretation. For this reason, we should never assume that specific types of dream imagery represent the same message for different children—or even for the same child over time. For example, in Olivia's case, her nightmare involving being chased by wolves may have initially started as a representation of her fear of dogs. By the time she got to my office years later, however, that nightmare had grown and transformed into something that made her relate to feeling she needed supernatural protection. Only the patient herself could have explained this and interpreted it to make sense for her.

DAYDREAMS
Dreams at night represent a way for the subconscious to communicate on a metaphorical level, such as occurred with Olivia when she was eight, or with literal imagery arising from a child's experiences, such as in Jared's case. Hypnosis can also be used to evoke daydreams that allow the subconscious to express itself similarly.

One such technique involves teaching the child to imagine being in a green room, such as the one people sit in during television shows, just before they are interviewed. I explained this concept to eleven-year-old Ethan, who had trouble falling asleep because he was afraid of having nightmares.

"Once you're in the room, you can notice a door. A sign on the door will say either 'Enter' or 'Closed.' Once the door says 'Enter,' this will mean that your subconscious has prepared a scene for you behind the door that will teach you something important."

Ethan nodded. In this case, I chose to give a vague instruction regarding what the subconscious might reveal in order to allow it to express whatever it deemed most important for Ethan. With other patients I might have given a more specific instruction about the content of the scene, such as that it would provide a solution to a particular dilemma.

"Are you ready?" I asked.

"Sure," he said tentatively.

"OK. Go to the green room and let me know when you see the door."

"I see it."

"What does it say?"

"It says *Enter.*"

"Great," I responded. "Now you can go through the door. You can describe what you find behind it to me, or you can experience the whole scene quietly, and when you return to the green room, you can tell me what you learned."

"Should I go in now?"

"Absolutely."

Ethan kept his eyes closed as his face narrowed in apparent concentration. He was silent for a few moments and then opened his eyes and smiled.

"What did you experience?" I asked.

"I saw myself in outer space," he said. "I traveled from planet to planet all over the universe."

"Wow!" I exclaimed as I offered to high-five him. "You have a great imagination. What do you think it means?"

He pondered a bit. "When I was traveling in the universe, I had two thoughts." He looked a bit perplexed. "They rhymed."

"What were the thoughts?

"The first one was 'When times are cruel and unfair, light will prevail, and I will be there.'"

"That's amazing," I said. "What do you think this means?"

"I think it means that my ancestors will be there to protect me."

Once again I was awed by the profound nature of a child's subconscious revelation. "And what was the other thought?"

"When all you see is black and gray, light will come and guide the way."

It seems that Ethan's subconscious was using the daydream to provide him with reassurance about his fears. I was reasonably certain that his self-therapy in this fashion was more effective for him than any reassurance that I might have given.

SEARCHING FOR MEANING

After many years of using hypnosis, I've learned to remain humble about my ability to correctly predict the issue that may underlie a particular symptom. For this reason, rather than making a guess about an issue, I view my job as facilitating my patients' process of figuring out what might be bothering them.

Zoe was referred to me at the age of sixteen because she suffered from anxiety and insomnia. She was able to fall asleep easily enough but woke up multiple times a night. She had complex family and social issues, and we worked through these over several weeks. Her anxiety improved a great deal, but her insomnia did not.

I told her there must be some psychological issue we had not yet dealt with and proposed using hypnosis to figure it out.

Zoe was enthusiastic about this suggestion, as she had proven herself to be gifted at the use of hypnosis.

"Why don't you imagine that you are in a movie theater?" I suggested. "You can imagine the comfortable seats that can recline back and even eating wonderful buttery popcorn."

"Got it," she said as she closed her eyes.

"Now, on the movie screen you will see yourself falling asleep. Then you will see yourself waking up at night. Please pay attention to the thoughts in your mind just before you wake up, so we can figure out what is bothering you."

"OK," she said softly. "I see myself falling asleep. Now I see my cat coming into the room and waking me up. I throw it off the bed, and then I go back to sleep. Now my cat comes back and wakes me again. I push it off the bed and go back to sleep. Then it wakes me up again."

She opened her eyes.

"Did you know your cat was waking you up?" I asked.

"No," she said. "That's weird."

"Where does your cat usually sleep?

"In my sister's room."

"So, close your bedroom door before you go to bed," I suggested.

The insomnia resolved immediately thereafter. And I learned that the subconscious can also help identify and resolve problems in the physical world.

WHAT YOU CAN DO ON YOUR OWN

Children have always had nightmares and will continue to do so. These abstract expressions of their fears and frustrations are a normal, healthy part of development. When nightmares become severe or recurring, though, there are ways you can help your child interpret them and get back to a normal sleep schedule. The first of these is by offering a gentle reality check on irrational fears (without demeaning them). For example, if your child has nightmares about someone breaking into your home, talk about how statistically unlikely that is to happen, let your child help lock doors at bedtime, and point out any other features of your family or home that help keep them safe (like a dog who would never let a stranger enter without making a fuss).

A second tool you can use to help kids work through nightmares is to help them determine how dreams end on their own terms—creating "Choose Your Own Adventure"-type scenarios. Encourage children to flip their fears by imagining endings that are silly or ironic or soothing. For example, the home invader in the aforementioned nightmare turns out to be a favorite cartoon character, a monster turns out to be made of peanut butter, or a child who dreams of being lost or alone discovers their pesky but beloved grandma follows along in every dream carrying snacks and a fuzzy sweater just in case she's needed. The specific scenario isn't important as long as it's comforting to the child. By examining dreams in this way, kids can begin to learn to put them in perspective and feel some control over how they feel about them.

Lastly, sometimes having a talisman to repel dreams works wonders for young children. Depending on your child's age, introducing a new stuffed animal, a special blanket presumed to have the power of invisibility, or a dream catcher near the bed can help. In each case, the object serves as an extension of your child's imagination, allowing them to create safe zones by harnessing their own creativity with just a little help from the props you provide.

The Lies We Tell Ourselves

How the Subconscious Can Help Us Become More Honest with Ourselves

We all practice self-deception sometimes—it's part of human nature, a tool we use to get along with others, to feel better, or to make things easier on ourselves. For example, it is easier for a child to feel she cannot go to school because of a stomachache than to recognize that she is afraid of a class bully. Another child might blame his teacher for not explaining the homework assignment clearly rather than dealing with his difficulty in understanding the subject matter. Engaging the subconscious within a trusting physician-patient relationship can shed light on problems that arise out of these denials and misconceptions and open pathways to acceptance and healing.

One of the most persistent cases of self-destructive denial I've treated was the struggle of a twelve-year-old boy whose family sought help for his behavioral tics. Liam might have initially presented as a child with a respiratory problem, because his first troublesome symptom was constantly clearing his throat after recovering from a bad cold. By the time I met him, though, he'd been through months of throat clearing, followed by months of frequently rotating and jerking his neck (to the point that his back hurt all the time), and then he'd returned to throat clearing again. He'd taken muscle relaxants, vitamins, and supplements, but the tics continued. In the sixth month after the problems started, Liam developed a stutter for the first time in his life. His entire family—mom, dad, and younger brother—were upset by this troubling trajectory.

Liam chose to sit in the furthest corner of my office from my own chair and to ask his mom to please remain in the waiting room. When I asked about his symptoms, Liam's stutter made it difficult for him to answer. He'd choose a way to explain the problem to me and then, after getting hung up on a word, choose a different approach (and a different first word). This is an adaptation many long-term stutters use to help them express themselves, but one they usually take some time to master. I guessed Liam was an intelligent and creative young man to have so quickly figured out an effective workaround.

I told him I believed he could learn to control his tics with hypnosis. Wanting to be clear about what he should expect, I further suggested that Liam might benefit from identifying whatever stressors might be related to his troubles. If there was an underlying problem, acknowledging it and dealing with it would help keep his behavior issues from coming back.

"When something is bothering you deep down," I explained, "it can keep bubbling up in different ways. Some kids develop headaches or stomachaches, and other kids become nervous or even develop tics and stuttering. The curious thing is that many times kids don't even realize that something is bothering them because it's buried inside their subconscious. Once they figure out what's wrong, they can fix it!"

At his next appointment, after learning how to use positive words and a hypnotic relaxation technique through imagining a sugar-white Caribbean beach, Liam told me he hadn't noticed any throat clearing or stuttering since I'd seen him last. This was surprising, as his mother told me his symptoms were still occurring all the time.

Why would Liam deny his symptoms? I asked whether he would let me communicate with his subconscious, which might be able to help us figure out what was going on, and he agreed.

SURPRISING ADVICE

When I explain communicating with the subconscious for the first time to a new patient, I offer a few standard instructions. Normally we begin with simple ideomotor signaling, so the first order of business is determining what the movement of each finger means (*Yes, No, I don't know,* or *I don't want to say*). Next I tell the patient I will ask the subconscious three important questions that will guide our progress:

1. *Are you willing to help the patient?* Usually the response is "yes." In the rare instance that the answer is "no," I will ask the subconscious some clarifying questions about its reluctance to help, including "Does the subconscious not know how to help the patient?" and "Does the subconscious think that the patient should solve the problem on his or her own?" Infrequently we identify that the subconscious is unavailable to help because of its preoccupation in dealing with its own problems. Sometimes we get around this hurdle when I ask, "If you knew how to help the patient, would you be willing to do so?"

2. *Is there something bothering the patient of which he or she is unaware?* If the answer is "yes," we might explore this issue at some point. At the start of our relationship, though, we don't make a commitment one way or the other.

3. *Do you have any advice for the patient?* If the subconscious answers "yes," then I suggest it share the advice with the patient. Sometimes this advice comes in the form of words or images, but at other times it may be communicated through feelings. If the answer is "no," I ask whether the subconscious would be willing to think up some advice it could share so that the patient can learn how to better interact with and learn from his or her subconscious. Usually, when we get to this stage, the subconscious ends up providing advice.

Liam was fine with all of this and said he was ready to get to work. His subconscious indicated that there was something bothering him of which he was unaware. When I asked the subconscious whether it had any advice, the subconscious indicated it did.

"Please share your advice with Liam," I said.

It's always up to the child whether to share this information with me. Liam didn't hesitate. He was eager to tell me what his subconscious had said and confused about how to handle it.

Looking at me with concern in his eyes, he shared this advice: *Stop being mean to other people.*

Liam was quick to follow this up by telling me, "I *am* nice."

I didn't doubt this was true but asked whether he could think of any relationship in which he might have been unkind. After some reflection, Liam said that sometimes he was mean to his brother, especially in the context of games they'd play together in which Liam, being four years older, had an advantage.

"I never thought about it," he said. "Is it weird that my subconscious says I should improve my behavior?"

I told him I thought his subconscious wanted him to be happy and healthy and that perhaps this was an important step. After all, the relationship between siblings is an important one. I suggested he practice deliberate kindness with his brother.

As he left that day, I walked Liam to the lobby, shook his hand, and told him, "It's great that you're able to be honest enough with yourself to allow the subconscious to give you that advice." I was serious. If Liam had been trying to hide or continue being hard on his brother, there's a good chance he would not have processed the advice, and he certainly wouldn't share it with me. This was a child who wanted to do better and feel better.

PLAYING NICE

Three weeks later, Liam's stuttering had improved, but his throat clearing remained unchanged. We discussed that he could lock up his tics in a treasure chest and throw it into the ocean off the beach in his relaxing place.

He said he'd been nicer to his brother, so he'd expected his problems to improve. However, when we went through the process of hypnosis again and he asked his subconscious for advice, it said he was too aggressive with his brother and that sometimes he hurt him when they played war games.

Liam reported all of this immediately, again with surprise. He'd done better, he said. He'd said nice things and taken turns.

I recommended engaging his brother in play that was less competitive and violent than playing war to see how that helped his problem. Maybe they could shoot their Nerf guns at targets instead of each other, or play soccer or cards, or build something together.

It would be another six weeks of slow, steady improvement in Liam's symptoms and resolute disagreement from his subconscious about how well he was treating his brother before the day arrived when Liam, his mother, and his subconscious all reported that he'd been kind and fair. At that time, his stuttering and throat clearing came to an end. The coincident resolution of both his physical symptoms and improvement in the sibling relationship suggested that Liam's tics and stuttering may have served as an expression of his difficulties with his brother. The two likely were intertwined. Perhaps this is why, initially, Liam believed his physical symptoms had improved when they had not, just as he believed his relationship with his brother was better when it was not. Until his sibling relationship had improved, his physical manifestations persisted.

I was struck that on three separate occasions Liam said he was acting appropriately, while his subconscious disagreed. Prior to this experience, I believed that a child who fails to report what they've done wrong is likely making a deliberate choice to lie. Liam's case was inconsistent with that theory. Made aware of the problem, he promised to work harder and told me he had—even when he undoubtedly knew his subconscious would tell the truth. Since he honestly told me repeatedly that his subconscious contradicted him (an inconsistency he could have withheld) and chose to seek ongoing guidance and act on it, I concluded that Liam was likely telling the truth as he consciously perceived it. He believed he was treating his brother fairly, and prior to invoking his subconscious, he had suppressed his awareness of the altercations with his brother, which contradicted that perspective.

TRUE LIES

In the years since meeting Liam, I've met other children who seem to have skewed views of the truth. Undoubtedly this is sometimes a deliberate effort to protect a secret, but many times it's clear the child holds a biased or incomplete memory or interpretation. Other children also suffered from physical manifestations of their stress over these deceptions.

The question, of course, is why. This takes us into territory where some things are unknown. Given two of the truths I've found to be consistent in the subconscious of almost every child I've treated with hypnosis—that the subconscious is both wise and loyal to the child—it's possible Liam's subconscious stepped into the role of conscience when Liam began to suffer physical symptoms because of his guilty feelings. This was his inner Jiminy Cricket letting him know something needed to change.

In many ways, feelings are the unique province of subconscious communication, a way to hint to the conscious person that something is happening that requires their attention. Liam's tics and his stutter may have been one step up from that—physical manifestations of unresolved feelings. Incomplete truth telling is common in childhood, but so is the confusion of emotions. Children (and adults, for that matter) may start to cry before they've fully processed that something is making them sad. They may act aggressively while still feeling happy during play, because they haven't gotten a handle on how to deal with something that makes them feel angry. And they may, like Liam, live with an imperfect relationship with the truth while they work out what about a situation is untenable for them.

PROTECTING PRIVILEGED INFORMATION

There are lots of reasons a patient might not want a parent to participate in a therapy session. The child may want to further his independence. She may have a secret she's not ready to share. He may feel the parent will judge his symptom or concern or even decide to intervene despite the child's wishes for the issue to be left alone. Some children make this choice deliberately, and others, like Liam, may not even know they're hiding a relevant truth. This is one reason I always ask children if they want to invite their parents to their sessions.

This is not something that only happens in the context of psychological problems. Denial is tricky that way. It can get in the way of any type of therapy, and it can also be a necessary coping mechanism the patient uses to protect him- or herself. I see patients every week for issues that are difficult to talk about—things like bedwetting, family discord, and potentially embarrassing behavioral issues. Many patients need time, circling around those issues, building trust, before they're ready to talk about them. Parents and clinicians alike need to respect the fact that breaking through the facade of denial is only helpful if the child finds a different way to cope with the problem. Otherwise it can do more harm than good.[1]

The help of Liam's subconscious and an unrushed therapy approach allowed him to face his problem a little at a time, as he was ready to deal with it. This could have gone any number of other ways. Liam could have continued to mistreat his brother until their relationship frayed for the long term. He could have ignored the signs that something was wrong and continued to live with tics that were disruptive and isolating. He could have been on a path to some future incident that would leave him branded as an abusive brother and with lingering guilt about his behavior.

Instead, his subconscious gently guided him to recognize and correct his behavior before the problem got out of hand. As a physician, I, too, have a responsibility to work with children at their own pace, and interacting with the subconscious routinely gives me good guidance on when and how to align with this timing.

Cases like Liam's can lead to the rare situation in which I recommend a parent leave a session (even if the child does not specifically request it). The reason I make this recommendation is simple: the subconscious might want to bring up an issue that the child doesn't want the parent to find out about. For example, it could be that the child has done something and is not ready to confess to a parent, wants to protect a parent from getting upset, or fears how the parent might try to "fix" the problem for them. Regardless of the reason, unless there's a danger to the child, the patient should have the opportunity to learn and consider whatever truth the subconscious has to share without the worry of how that same secret might be received by someone else. If the subconscious is holding it back, chances are the child needs time to digest it. In fact, sometimes in therapy the subconscious will explicitly indicate, in speech or writing, that the child is not ready to face that truth. It may even help map out gradual steps to help the child understand and cope with the sensitive material.

Many times in my work with patients who engage the subconscious during hypnosis therapy, we reach a point at which the subconscious directs the child, "Tell the rest" or "Tell the truth," and the child then feels ready to do so. These are breakthrough moments that allow children to begin making peace with their problems and eventually move on from them.

WHAT YOU CAN DO ON YOUR OWN

Liam's case teaches us that patients sometimes truly fail to recall uncomfortable events in their lives consciously and that these may be accessible through interaction with the subconscious. When a child denies something has occurred, parents should not assume the child is lying. Instead, consider helping your child quiet his or her conscious mind and encourage closer examination of the problem. Consider it a positive, proactive take on the parental admonishment "I want you to think about what you've done."

Hypnosis is a highly effective way to quiet the mind, but there are also things you can encourage children to do at home:

- Deliberate breathing: The simple act of slowing down and thinking about one's breathing, focusing on inhaling slowly through the nose and exhaling slowly through the mouth, has an immediate calming effect. Even with no other intervention, children (and adults) can benefit from turning their attention inward, to breath coming in and going out, to recenter themselves.
- Getting outside: Turns out the age-old parenting directive to go outside and play has identifiable, measurable benefits. Among them are the power of a change of venue from inside to outside to interrupt stressful and negative thought loops. Some of this is undoubtedly attributable to the environmental change: different light, air, sounds, and smells. Some of it may also go back to a deep genetic connection human beings have with the natural world.[2]
- Bringing nature in: Playing nature sounds, looking at live plants, or watching fish swim in a tank can all help kids feel more relaxed and less stressed. It's no coincidence that my offices feature a giant fish tank or that most kids choose personal relaxing places to visit in hypnosis that are outside.
- Talk about it: Prompt your child with honest curiosity and respect rather than admonitions. Rather than saying, "How could you do such a terrible thing?" you might ask, "Please tell me what you were thinking that led you to make that choice." Teenagers often respond that they were not thinking or that they did not consider all of the alternatives. You can ask for their input about how they might think things out more carefully in the future, such as through quieting their minds and listening to their own subconscious wisdom.

16

The World According to John, Amy, and Elise

The Fruits of Treating the Subconscious with Respect, Kindness, and Acceptance

Developing a basic understanding of the characteristics of the subconscious in no way undermines its ability to surprise and amaze. I frequently meet complex and complicated iterations of the inner advisor, including some with personalities so divergent from what I can see in the patient they inhabit that it challenges the mind to understand where they are coming from. These subconscious forms sometimes possess and share knowledge seemingly unknown to either the patient or the patient's family and that they might even deny. Over time, I've learned that carefully and respectfully considering any information the subconscious offers—even if I have to set aside my own preconceptions—can be instrumental in helping almost any child heal.

More often than not, a child's subconscious seems like a center of calm within, a resource they can draw on once they learn how to tap into its advice and knowledge. It's easy for kids to envision this entity as a miniature version of themselves, but I'd argue a typical subconscious is better described as a more mature and more clear-eyed version of the conscious self. This is not surprising, considering the overarching role the subconscious plays in each person's life. As I explain to my patients, even though the subconscious is the part of their minds they're usually not aware of, it is nevertheless a big part of who they are, and a busy one! For example, the subconscious regulates the body's breathing while we are awake and asleep. The subconscious coordinates the movement of all the parts of our anatomy when we chew or walk or give a thumbs-up. The subconscious stores our memories, keeping them at the ready or just out of reach or deeply buried.

The subconscious also helps manage our thoughts and feelings, and sometimes this creates conflict between subconscious and conscious thought, leading to confused emotions or even the development of physical or psychological symptoms. For example, a child with a fraught relationship with a "frenemy" may begin to feel dizzy or nauseous when around that person, or a child may say (and believe) he feels "fine," even as his eyes fill with tears. As physical symptoms manifest, children may begin to grasp emotions that have been roiling beneath the surface of conscious thought, perhaps for a long time.

In one common scenario in which the subconscious can help children sort out their problems, a child presents with symptoms that suggest a physical disorder but are actually being caused by something psychological. This can be as small a thing as a headache or a stomachache that crops up when the child feels anxious. But these children can also be terribly sick—so ill they can end up heavily medicated or hospitalized. That was the case with a teenage patient named John who'd been sick to his stomach and experiencing severe bone and joint pain for months.[1] John dropped forty pounds and lost consciousness several times before I met him. He was in the hospital then, bone-thin in his pajamas, with dark circles under his eyes. I arrived at the same time as his dinner tray and noted that he looked at it with disgust without even lifting the lid to see what was on it. John was seventeen years old, and by his own assessment, he was nervous about everything. This alone could not begin to explain how poorly he'd been doing, though, and he'd undergone a barrage of invasive medical tests (rightly so, considering his severe symptoms) that hadn't turned up any evidence of disease.

Consciously, John did not want to be sick. He certainly didn't want to be in pain all the time or vomiting every day or passing out at school. When I suggested maybe his subconscious could help us get to the bottom of what was happening to him, he quickly agreed to learn how to communicate with it through typing. It took only a few minutes of interaction with John's subconscious to ascertain that a deeply felt emotional crisis was behind his illness—not any kind of physical disease. John's subconscious told me that John was gay, that he was having a hard time accepting this about himself, and that his mother had told him flat out that if he was gay, she would throw him out of the house.

This was a young man struggling to accept himself, all the while knowing that the most important person in his life at that time would *not* accept him. Somewhere in his psyche, he'd recognized this as an impossible situation, and his deeply held insecurities and conflict had begun to emerge in the form of pain, nausea, and sickness.

John's case was extreme, both in terms of the severe form his physical symptoms took and in the challenges he faced because his family was unsupportive (and borderline threatening). But the phenomenon of converting one kind of pain to another is a common one. In fact, most of us experience it at some point—when a headache prevents a child from taking a dreaded test or a physical symptom we've learned to live with most of the time seems intolerable when we're stressed out or angry.

One critical aspect of conversion of a mental process to a physical symptom, as with denial (chapter 15), is that if it's happening, it's happening for a reason. In small things (like the headache that comes on before a test), recognizing the connection often leads to an opportunity to address the cause on a conscious level, at which point the symptom ceases. For example, recurrent headaches can resolve once we discuss how to study more effectively for tests and thus decrease the associated dread. In complex cases like John's, though, his physical symptoms were the only way he was "dealing with" his extreme inner conflict and anxiety. They were a defense mechanism his subconscious mind created to protect him because the underlying issues were too overwhelming to resolve on a conscious level. Before helping him let that defense mechanism go, I had to be sure he could cope with the feelings he'd experience without it.

In this, too, I relied on help from John's subconscious, which guided John to process his feelings a little at a time on a conscious level. This provided him with his first opportunity to acknowledge his sexual orientation without being judged. It was during work with his doctor rather than with his family, but it was a start, and his physical symptoms began to abate.

We've all heard jesting speculation that mothers have eyes in the backs of their heads. John's case demonstrates how, in some ways, the subconscious is the closest thing to this—a kind of observer who sees and knows everything that's going on in our bodies and minds. And just like a good mom, a vigilant and helpful subconscious can give us perspective and guidance when things aren't going well.

THE SYMPTOM IS THE SOLUTION

While situations involving denial do not always cause development of physical symptoms, by definition conversion disorders always involve development of a physical symptom that typically offers a solution for a patient's difficult psychological conflict.[2] In John's case, his nearly life-threatening symptoms may have reflected his self-rejection.

In another example of conversion, for three weeks thirteen-year-old Aniya developed constant difficulty breathing related to vocal cord dysfunction. This problem occurred even while she slept, which is very unusual for a functional symptom that typically resolves during sleep. Thus, her symptom was more consistent with a diagnosis of conversion disorder. Her subconscious explained in typing that she had seen her stepfather smoking weed and did not want this fact disclosed to her mother, for fear of disrupting the marriage. The subconscious then typed, "I can't let her talk about it." I helped Aniya overcome her symptom by suggesting to her that she could learn to trust herself.[3]

Connor, a healthy seventeen-year-old who loved playing basketball, fell while playing, hit his head against a wall, and lost consciousness. When he recovered a few moments later, he complained of a headache, lower back pain, and an inability to walk. A medical workup did not reveal a cause of the paralysis of his legs, and it was suspected that he might have developed a conversion disorder. As is typical of such patients, Connor said he was unaware of any psychological issue that could have led to development of his symptom (if he had been aware of the issue, he likely would not have developed the physical symptom). Nonetheless, his subconscious explained that Connor was conflicted because his girlfriend had threatened to leave him if he kept playing so much basketball and did not pay sufficient attention to her. Thus, his inability to walk reflected his paralysis about how to balance his love of the sport with his love of his girlfriend. He recovered once he learned how to better balance his life tasks.[4]

A CALL FOR HELP

Sometimes a child's subconscious takes an unexpected form. One of my young patients, an eleven-year-old boy, heard his subconscious speak in the voice of the grandfather who'd died when he was just four years old. In fact, he felt his grandfather had been guiding him all his life. Another patient imagined a relaxing place from a bygone era and believed her subconscious took the form of a historical figure from that past.

Even though the inner advisor of each of these patients brought surprises, each ultimately stayed true to the most important characteristics of the subconscious: having the child's best interest at heart and being willing to help them work through critical issues during hypnosis.

One case that taught me a great deal arose during the treatment of a sixteen-year-old girl. She had a long and complex medical history that included major surgery, a childhood stroke, neurological difficulties, severe headaches, and anxiety. I worked with Amy on a few occasions over three years to teach her how she could use hypnosis to cope with her various health challenges.

And then, in what seemed a desperate bid for help, Amy went to her school in the middle of the night with a razor and dialed 911, informing the operator she might hurt someone. After she was evaluated at a psychiatric facility and discharged, I met with Amy and asked what had happened. She told me she'd heard a deep voice telling her to hurt herself.

"It told me to walk to the high school," she said.

"Had you ever heard this voice before?"

"No."

"Is it still there?" I asked.

"No."

"How did you think of calling 911?" I wondered.

"Well," she said in a tone that suggested this answer was obvious, "I thought the police should know."

Of course, she was right. This was excellent thinking.

During hypnosis and using ideomotor signaling, Amy was able to communicate with her subconscious, and one of the first things she told me was that its name was Andrew. In addition, she described her soul as having gone "to sleep" after her stroke.

I was surprised to learn that Amy's subconscious did not share her gender but not surprised to realize she had such a complex inner life. This is usually the case with children who've dealt with severe and long-term physical or mental health problems. I believe that the subconscious's efforts to help a child by necessity reflect the complex nature of their physical or mental health problems. However, I have observed that in some patients, conflicts at the subconscious level can lead to the persistence of their symptoms.

I have since met many children who've discovered their subconscious does not share their gender. Sometimes this is a notable factor in their treatment, and sometimes it is not. In Amy's case, it eventually became clear that this facet of her inner advisor directly linked to an internal struggle she'd been dealing with for years: Amy identified as a boy. This child was transgender but just beginning to think about how to incorporate that critical facet of identity into her life. Amy had been afraid to talk about this feeling and in fact did not know how to explain it for a long time. Since meeting Amy, I've worked with nine other transgender individuals. In each case, the subconscious identified with a gender other than the birth gender. Overall, however, about 10 percent of my patients' subconscious voices identify as the opposite gender of the child, and the majority of these children are not transgender.

It may seem surprising to have two successive cases come along in which the subconscious reveals a hidden facet of a teen's personality—in one a boy's sexual orientation and in the other a teen's gender identity—but these are heavy issues for teens to grapple with. The paths they take from being children who seek to have their identities defined for them to becoming adults who are comfortable and confident in who they need to be are often marked with difficult, emotional hurdles. In each of these cases, however, the subconscious helped the child clear an obstacle and move further down that track. In Amy's case, once her family understood the root of the conflict that had been causing her so much anxiety and pain, they supported her transition. They welcomed their transformed child with the name he chose and his new gender expression.

A GIRL AND HER GHOST

Of the many subconscious interactions I've had with children, few have had higher stakes or a more hopeful outcome than that of a young girl who addressed my questions with deadly serious intent. Elise was twelve years old when she was referred to me by her pediatrician for anxiety, but it was apparent from our first meeting that anxiety was the least of her problems. This was a girl in crisis. At an age when she should have been just beginning to shift her worldview from that of a child to that of an adolescent, she had already twice attempted suicide and ended up in psychiatric hospitals. She was experiencing hallucinations, including one of a ghost who came to her every night to tell her she should kill herself. She had been prescribed a number of different psychiatric drugs, and their combined effects included making her so tired and lethargic she found it difficult to think.

I often meet patients I recognize immediately as being prime candidates for hypnosis therapy, kids I feel confident I can help—and teach to help themselves in the long term. This was not one of these cases. This was a little girl on a precipice, and I hoped I could help her.

Elise was able to learn hypnosis quickly and allowed her subconscious to communicate through typing. Whether the subconscious knows if something is bothering the child, whether it knows what the problem is, and whether it will share that information with me or the patient are all routine questions in hypnosis therapy, but when I asked what was bothering Elise, her subconscious's response was not typical. I sat and watched with quiet concern as her fingers typed without pause or interruption for nearly twenty-five minutes, generating four single-spaced pages of notes. The juxtaposition of her youth and the hyper-focused report her subconscious was creating about what was wrong in her life was jarring, especially when she finally put her hands down, emerged from hypnosis, and reported that she neither remembered making nor wanted to read the list.

With her permission, I reviewed it. It depicted a strained relationship with her father. It detailed bullying at school. It described a betrayal by a friend. It said she hated taking so many medications and feeling different and like an outsider all the time. It said she was afraid of the ghost and of what it kept telling her to do.

I tell my patients that even in the face of our most complicated and serious problems, the best we can do is start by taking one positive step, and then another. One of my favorite quotes to share with kids is from Lao Tzu, who wrote, "A journey of a thousand miles must begin with a single step." With this in mind, I told Elise that each time I saw her from then on, we would work together on one of the items on her list.

If I had known how important the ghost would turn out to be in Elise's therapy, we would have started with it, but since it was the fifth item on the list her subconscious made, we didn't discuss it again until her fifth session after the typing that had given us so much to work on.

When I asked whether the ghost was still coming every night, Elise said it was.

"And does it still want you to kill yourself?" I asked.

"Yes."

"Do you know why?"

"No."

After thinking about this idea for a bit and sticking with the approach of meeting patients where they were, I told her I'd like to speak to the ghost.

"How could you do that?" she asked.

"Ask it to come here, and then you can tell me what it says."

Elise looked at me as if I'd lost my mind. "I can't ask her to come," she said. "She only comes *at night*."

"I think you have more control here than you realize," I said. "Ask her to come."

The girl closed her eyes momentarily and then reopened them, looking surprised. "She's here."

"Good," I said. "Can you ask her if she would answer my questions?"

"She says yes."

"Great. Can you please ask her if it's true that she wants you to die?"

"She says it's true."

"Ask her why."

"She says I've had a horrible childhood. If I kill myself, I can relive it in a better way."

This was crazy logic, but it was logic, and I could follow it well enough to make a case against it.

"Please tell the ghost I appreciate that she wants to help you," I said. "Tell her I'm helping you deal better with your childhood now, one thing at a time, and that you've learned how to use hypnosis to feel better."

Elise nodded, apparently confirming that she was sharing my message, so I continued.

"I want you to tell your ghost that one day, when you die of old age, that's when you will choose whether to relive your childhood." I used *when* rather than *if* as a strong suggestion that this decision would not be influenced by the ghost.

I waited while Elise and her ghost processed this notion. Finally Elise said, "She says she's willing to let me help myself, and I don't need to kill myself. She would like to become my guardian angel instead."

"Would that be OK with you?" I asked.

"As long as I don't have to see her," Elise replied. Apparently she had seen her ghost enough for a lifetime.

Six months later, I discharged Elise from my care after helping her eliminate all but a single antidepressant from her medication regimen. She no longer had nightmares, no longer saw a ghost, no longer reported having urges toward self-harm, and was hopeful about the future. She was, after taking a terrible detour into a frightening level of instability, feeling like a kid with mostly normal tween problems. She owed much of her recovery to the subconscious, so incongruous with her personality, which had taken meticulous care to detail everything that was going wrong in her life. We hadn't banished all of her problems, but we'd been able to work together to find coping strategies and tools for her to deal with each of them in turn.

REASON TO BELIEVE

John, Amy, and Elise's stories inevitably prompt skepticism. After all, cooperating with a subconscious to help a teenager begin to deal with issues of sexual orientation or gender identity is unusual. Debating with a ghost about whether the continual haunting of a child is a useful strategy appears to presume an improbable "reality" at best. These three children are among many of my patients whose subconscious observations proved to be complicated and challenging to process. Inevitably, they engender questions: How do you know the subconscious is right?

How does a subconscious get a name—and a boy's name? Where does the conscious child end and the subconscious begin? How do you know it was the subconscious typing and not the child's conscious mind? Why would you ask the girl to summon the ghost?

All these questions have essentially the same answer: when offered an unexpected, unlikely, or even otherworldly scenario in the course of treating a child, in almost every case I choose to take the child (and the child's subconscious) at his or her word. If a child believes something to be true, my best chance of being able to help that child is to accept his or her assumptions as true and work from there. The patient needs to be heard and understood. Starting from a place of distrust weakens my connection with these children, so I don't do it.

And why would I? In the case of the patient who believes his dead grandfather's spirit is part of his subconscious, the child finds an important and powerful ally in that manifestation (or actual presence, whichever is the case). What would be gained by questioning or meddling in that empowering dynamic when it is helping my patient to heal? In Amy's case, identifying (or recognizing, depending on your perspective) her subconscious as male helped her begin a long and long-overdue journey toward self-realization and acceptance. In Elise's case, speaking with the ghost she believed was driving her toward suicide gave either her or the ghost (or both) the means and motivation to stop having that conversation. Whether the ghost was real, a figment of Elise's imagination, a metaphor for her fears, a part of her personality, and/or some form of her subconscious really doesn't matter as long as my interactions with the ghost helped her heal.

WHAT YOU CAN DO ON YOUR OWN

The major cases in this chapter were all ones in which it was obvious the child needed professional help. But sometimes that need is not so obvious. There are always actions you can take at home to help your child, but there are also times when the most important thing you can do is recognize that those attempts are not enough. A parent often is

the most qualified observer to recognize whether a child needs professional intervention, but many are nevertheless unsure about whether or
when to ask for help. This dilemma doesn't represent a failing; on the
contrary, it means parents are thinking deeply about how to proceed in
the best interest of their children. Parents of children with chronic and
severe illnesses may face some of the most difficult of these dilemmas.
They often have to figure out not only whether a situation is abnormal
but also whether it is too abnormal to manage independently of the
health care system. As a parent, I have faced these decisions too, and
even with a medical degree and decades of experience treating patients,
I've sometimes found it daunting and wondered who was going to help
my child. With that in mind, I recommend asking yourself the following
questions if you're unsure about whether you should seek professional
help. If you're still in doubt, err on the side of caution and consult
a medical professional you trust. Your child's pediatrician or family
medicine provider is an excellent place to start.

- *Is this a serious problem?* This may sound obvious, but it is very common for relatively small issues to get blown out of proportion and also
  for large ones to be ignored. I often remind my patients to abide by
  the five-by-five rule: don't spend more than five minutes on anything
  that won't matter in five years. Parents should consider this as well.
  Things like your child's nail biting or your teen's nose ring or a behavioral tic that crops up but doesn't do any harm may be disconcerting
  in the short term, but if you look at them from a bird's-eye view, most
  problems become manageable, and most work themselves out.
- *What are the potential consequences?* Hand in hand with the five-by-
  five guideline is the question of consequence. Children often choose
  to assert themselves or express their personalities through quirky
  choices—perhaps by changing their appearance, or adopting dietary
  restrictions, or trying out new personality facets that aren't very
  agreeable to the rest of family. These can be harmless experiments.
  The true test is in how they're playing out. Has the child who has

changed appearance also stopped taking care of himself or doing his schoolwork? Has the child with a new diet lost weight? Is that new personality colored by anger or despair that doesn't resolve itself in a short time? Is there any talk of feeling worthless or of self-harm? All these signs merit seeking help from a professional.

- *Is there an obvious reason?* Difficult life moments require us to make adjustments, and this is just as true for children as it is for adults. If your child is going through a hardship like a divorce or death in the family, a change in health status, a move, or a school change, some anxiety or unhappiness may be par for the course. It's OK to give your child a little time to get used to a new normal, but if you feel the circumstances are more than they can handle, or if your child's emotions do not rebalance within a few weeks, ask for help.

- *What does my child think?* While there are certainly children and teens who work to minimize their worries, most children are able to help gauge their own need for help. Amy was a perfect example: calling 911 on herself got the ball rolling toward an intervention in her emotional crisis. If you are concerned, ask your child whether he or she would like to talk with someone outside the family who will respect their privacy and help them sort out their feelings.

IV

THE POWER OF THE SPIRIT

This Life of Mine

Shifting toward Self-Determination

Novelist Alice Walker wrote, "The most common way people give up their power is by thinking they don't have any." Her words speak to an essential and all-too-common issue children face: they are dependents who often feel powerless to control their own circumstances. They generally don't control where they live, what school they attend, whether or when they see a doctor, or even what's for dinner. For children who live with chronic physical and mental health problems, this issue is amplified as parents, teachers, and health care providers take necessary steps to guide and protect them. Frequently, those same adults take extra steps as well, helping and managing kids' lives more than is necessary. These well-meaning actions may further urge children toward passive attitudes—outlooks that do nothing to help them learn to become independent, active patients and effective advocates for their own needs.

One of the most crucial facets of hypnosis therapy—perhaps the single most important—is that because kids learn how to help heal themselves with its use, it gives them a sense of their own power. The implications of that impact are wide ranging. Children gain confidence; they begin to fully grasp that the world doesn't just happen *to* them; they take ownership of their symptoms, their treatments, and how they choose to perceive and handle challenges. Many times it becomes apparent that they can manage even problems that seem insurmountable.

Encouragingly, this impact is not only among the most important outcomes of hypnosis therapy but also widely achieved.

Over the course of my career, I've spoken with parents, teachers,
physicians, and former patients who've been kind enough to commend
my work with hypnosis. From the very beginning, however, it's been apparent to me that the "magic" of any healing, confidence, and maturity
my patients achieve comes from within. My job (and that of any hypnosis practitioner who wants to facilitate long-term positive results) is
to help children identify and bring out skills and talents that are already
within them.

As is the case with so many aspects of my understanding of hypnosis,
I first recognized this fact while I was treating Paul.

Paul was a young man who had lived in fear of his medical condition
all his life and often felt like a victim of it, powerless to control his fate. I
would have given anything to be able to cure him of his life-threatening
allergies, but even today modern medicine has not created a solution
to his medical problems (though we continue to get closer). At first, I
treated Paul's symptoms, medicated him, and helped him understand
the treatments and procedures that were necessary to keep him alive.
Those were all steps I could take as a pulmonologist to try to keep him
well.

When we began incorporating hypnosis into Paul's appointments,
however, the impact of his treatment took a dramatic turn. Paul learned
how to manage his own pain. He learned how to turn off the crippling
anxiety that had summoned asthma episodes that were virtually in-
distinguishable from those caused by actual allergens. He was able to
express and deal with his feelings and fears about living with a disease
that could kill him on any given day. He was able to calm himself at will,
even in incredibly stressful situations, by self-hypnotizing and going to
the center of the clear, quiet lake in his mind.

A feeling of health is relative. A good day for someone with chronic
breathing issues may simply be a day with no medical intervention—a
day when focus shifts from dealing with an illness to enjoying life. A

good day for a patient dealing with anxiety may be one of seemingly miniscule accomplishments—getting out of bed on time, going to school, keeping his or her private, crushing fears at bay from breakfast to bedtime. Many of my patients struggle with monumental physical and psychological issues. Recognizing and claiming even a small sense of control over their own circumstances is often the first step in whatever healing journey is uniquely possible for them.

PUTTING THE PATIENT IN THE DRIVER'S SEAT

In every patient encounter, I strive to demonstrate to the children in my care that they have power over their own health. It starts at hello, with my greeting the child first and then the parent, asking the child who will be attending the appointment, and waiting for the child to explain what's going on. Once we've talked about the problem, the first question about what to do next also goes to the child.

"Are you ready for us to discuss the ways hypnosis can help you?"

At every step throughout a child's care, I reinforce the fact that patients can be in charge of their own health.

As a medical doctor, this is perhaps the most important tenet I have carried over from the world of hypnosis, and it is a game changer. Consulting with rather than dictating to patients about what they want to do helps them feel ownership of their health issues and any solutions we can create. When I propose a treatment, if the child has a problem with it, we find out on day one in the office instead of months or even years later, when it turns out they haven't been taking a medication or doing a treatment because they don't like how it makes them feel or because they believe it's been forced on them. Patients who choose their own treatment plans—even if they only have two or three not-very-appealing options—are far more likely to follow through, to believe they can succeed, and to take responsibility if they see a need for change.[1] These are all positive, productive outcomes.

The same rules apply in teaching hypnosis. I explain that kids will remain in control and that they'll be in charge of using the tool in whatever way works best for them. They learn how to access the wisdom of their subconscious, and I encourage them to develop their own systems for relying on it when they need it. With the child's permission, I prompt the subconscious to help direct their therapy. Just as in every other facet of care, this presumes that children already possess power and knowledge to help heal themselves. Approaching patient care with this attitude builds trust and sets positive expectations for therapy. I've spoken with clinicians who actually aren't comfortable with this approach, worrying that if expectations aren't met, then kids will be disappointed. Personally (and professionally), I'd much rather deal with the consequences of unmet expectations—something I can frame as part of life's journey—while giving patients hope, confidence, and the will to make an effort that can propel them to their best possible outcome.

The scope of this approach and kids' efforts and outcomes vary a great deal depending on the diagnosis. Even with that caveat, I believe there is always room for hope and improvement, as demonstrated in the examples of Rae, Grace, and Eric.

RAE

Sometimes even a small shift in perspective can have a potentially life-changing impact.

Rae was ten when she moved near the hospital where I was director of the Pediatric Pulmonary and Cystic Fibrosis Center and became my patient. She was a tiny, dynamic girl, super smart for her age, and already making friends in her new school. Rae's diagnosis was cystic fibrosis, so she was very much in need of a lung specialist to monitor her treatment and guide her care. She came into my life in my earliest years of practicing hypnosis with patients, but even in those days, the positive results I was seeing made me feel that I had a medical responsibility to take the time to offer and teach it to any child who wanted to learn.

For patients suffering from lung disease, it doesn't take a significant leap of logic to recognize that any therapy that helps them relax at will has direct health benefits. Many kids who struggle to breathe understandably develop anxiety and even panic when they're short of breath. If their bodies respond by producing adrenaline, creating so-called fight-or-flight reactions, they can find it even more difficult to catch their breath and achieve calm.[2]

Rae was dealing with this issue on a regular basis. Both she and her parents assumed this frequent and distressing problem was an unavoid-able by-product of her disease. Because of it, she was leading a largely sedentary life—not a natural state for a school-aged child. The thing is, in an oddly chicken/egg scenario, it can be difficult to determine in cases like Rae's whether her anxiety was worsening her shortness of breath or whether her shortness of breath was causing her anxiety. Ei-ther way, she needed a tool she could use to feel more in control of both her stress and her breathing. When I asked whether she'd like to learn to use hypnosis to accomplish this result, she loved the idea of having a skill no one else in her class likely had.

Rae was an eager student, practicing hypnosis twice every day, mentally going to the relaxing place she'd chosen—a tent in the woods under a tree strung with fairy lights. Each time I saw her, she was eager to demonstrate how well she was doing, especially when she'd mastered achieving calm on command by crossing her fingers as her relaxation sign.

Rae's disease was indisputable, but it turned out that the symptom that had been keeping her benched from activities was mostly based in her anxieties, not in her cystic fibrosis. Within a few appointments, the shortness of breath that had been such a defining event in her days had largely disappeared.

A few weeks after learning to self-hypnotize, Rae was playing outside with her friends. In the second month, she signed up for a community soccer program. Each step was a great development for her physical and mental health. She had chosen a therapy, wholeheartedly embraced its practice, and managed to significantly improve her day-to-day life.

Putting this patient in the driver's seat was the first critical step in helping her to overcome her debilitating symptom. Before she could change the way she was experiencing it, she had to take ownership of it and believe she could make a difference.

GRACE

For patients who become accomplished at hypnosis, it's possible to "level up" as they learn to rely on their subconscious to help them. It never ceases to amaze me how much kids can accomplish when they're able to get in sync with this part of themselves that drives so many of their processes, emotions, and reactions. Seeking answers and guidance from within rather than from an outside source gives kids confidence; it allows them to think, *Somewhere deep inside, I know the answer. I know what to do.*

With many patients, I've been lucky enough to watch this internal partnership develop. One of the most memorable was Grace, a young lady whose use of hypnosis spanned many months and multiple health concerns.

Grace was a twenty-year-old college student studying environmental science when she first came to my office, referred by the pediatric oncologist who'd been overseeing her care through several years of cancer treatment, including two recurrences. Grace was enrolled in a promising new chemotherapy clinical trial, but the treatments were causing nausea and vomiting—symptoms so severe they were making her miserable and putting her participation at risk. She arrived at her appointment looking every inch the environmentally minded young woman. She wore scuffed hiking boots, sweatpants, and a faded Earth Day T-shirt under her flannel shirt. Her head was covered by a knit cap. She was cheerful, engaging, and surprisingly optimistic for someone I knew had been feeling very poorly. The deep blue-brown hollows ringing her eyes were the only hint of how much her treatment had strained her body.

Grace was skeptical about hypnosis, but, as she put it, she was willing to try anything. I told her I believed she could alter her perception of her nausea to overcome it—that other patients had successfully been

able to do this before her. Grace chose a beach in Antigua as her relaxing place and quickly learned to go there at will with hypnosis. Being
relaxed made her feel a little better, but it didn't counteract her nausea.
In talking about her treatments, she said she could only have small sips
of water on her chemotherapy infusion days and they never seemed like
enough. With that in mind, we devised the imagery of rainfall on her
beach as something Grace could envision when she felt ill. The rainfall
imagery was tied to relieving a different physical symptom—thirst—but
she made an association between not feeling thirsty and not feeling
nauseous. The suggestion worked, perhaps because imagery involving
falling liquid such as raindrops or waterfalls is a useful metaphor for
fluid going down, which counteracts nausea that involves a feeling of
fluid moving upward. She was able to tolerate her last several rounds of
treatment and finish the trial. In fact, at the end of it, she was the only
patient at our hospital to report *not* experiencing nausea.

Several months after her chemotherapy ended, Grace came back
because she was suffering from debilitating anxiety, insomnia, and
unexplained pain at the site where her tumor had been. I asked what
she thought would be more helpful: to figure out why she was anxious
or to figure out a way to relieve her anxiety without delving into the
cause. She said she wanted to know why. Taking this response to heart,
we agreed that it was time to consult with her subconscious. I taught
her how to type in hypnosis, and she prepared a list of questions she
wanted me to ask. As she returned to the mental relaxing place of her
beach in Antigua, she sat at one keyboard, and I sat at another. This is
a shortened version of the interaction that followed:

Q: Hello, am I talking to Grace's subconscious?

Grace: *Yes.*

Q: How are you feeling?

Grace: *Very relaxed.*

Q: Good. Grace wants to know why she has been so anxious lately?

Grace: *Nervous.*

Q: About what?

Grace: *Chemo and how it's really working.*

Q: Why is she more nervous than in the past?

Grace: *Because things are going good can it last?*

Q: Things have been too good?

Grace: *Health wise. Things are always going wrong usually. Infections, etc.*

Q: Please explain why Grace is so anxious now—she has been getting chemo for six years and hasn't been this anxious before.

Grace: *Maybe I'm tired of all this and now I just want to stop going through it all.*

Q: Who is tired of all this, you or Grace, or both?

Grace: *Both. We both would like to be healthy for a long period of time.*

Q: I think I understand. So let's see if we can help you: How do you think you should approach the uncertainty of your treatments in terms of attitude? What do you think would be the best attitude for Grace to adopt?

Grace: *A sort of take it as it comes type of attitude. Maybe a living for today sort of thing.*

Q: I agree. Can you help her let go of her wanting to plan for the future, and let her better adopt the attitude of living for today?

Grace: *Yes it should be easy.*

Q: So, please tell her these things, and help shape her attitude in the way you know is best.

Grace: *OK.*

Q: Has she accepted your suggestion?

Grace: *Yes.*

Q: Good. How does she feel?

Grace: *Very good about it.*

Q: Excellent. Now, tell me about Grace's pain. Why is she getting it?

Grace: *She gets worried and it irritates her nerves.*

Q: So do you think the pain will now be better because she has a new attitude?

Grace: *If she can stay relaxed and calm, she'll be fine.*

Q: Excellent. Now, tell me why she can't sleep well lately.

Grace: *Too many things on her mind . . . her brain is still going and she can't shut it off at night.*

Q: What can you or she do to help her sleep better?

Grace: *Clear her mind.*

Q: How can she do that?

Grace: *By relaxing and taking deep breaths.*

Q: Great. Has this session been helpful?

Grace: *Yes.*

Q: Will Grace remember?

Grace: *Yes.*

Q: Could you please allow her to feel very good about herself and about being able to solve her anxiety problem?

Grace: *Yes.*

Q: Great. So, after you have done that, please come on back.

It seemed that even though Grace's medical condition was stable, her insecurities about her cancer and her sense of being at its mercy persisted. After this session delving into the questions she wanted to ask her subconscious, she said that, as she'd been typing, she'd felt like she was observing herself but was saying things of which she was not conscious. When the session was over, she said she felt much better, with no pain at her tumor site and no anxiety.

The next time I saw Grace, she told me she'd used hypnosis every night for three weeks to fall asleep, and after that she hadn't needed it anymore. Sleep was her friend again.

Grace had successfully managed to interact with her subconscious and enlist it in actively helping her feel better. Over the years, I've seen many other patients accomplish this task, each in their own way. A few have learned to use ideomotor signaling to answer their own questions. One boy learned to have typed exchanges with his subconscious while he was in hypnosis. He would seek its counsel and then watch as his hands typed responses. After each of these self-directed sessions, he'd report that he felt better—even though he chose not to go back and read his transcripts.

Being able to consult their own inner advisor—to rely on it like an inner power—is one of children's most empowering benefits of hypnosis.

ERIC

Perhaps the children who benefit most from hypnosis are those who achieve a level of self-empowerment that lets them tap into their inner abilities at will. It gives them a deeply felt confidence even in troubled times, which supports the maturity to manage consequential plans and actions. This was the case with Eric, for whom hypnosis became an indispensable way of life during a difficult time.[3]

Sometimes the place where a child finds peace during hypnosis is close to home. That was certainly the case for Eric, a teen with a rare and severe lung disease. When I visited his family's house for his graduation party, I recognized the spot he'd been describing as his relaxing place for the two years we'd been working together: the lush, sloping yard; the small, white house in the distance; the stand of maple and birch trees. In hypnosis, Eric said it smelled like freshly mowed grass.

The sun was always streaming down, warm and white, shining on him, passing through his body, lighting the diseased corners of his lungs and healing them.

Eric's condition had dictated limitations over most aspects of his young life. He hadn't been able to physically exert himself, because playing tag or running or even climbing a flight of stairs left him winded and exhausted. Prolonged steroid treatment had limited his growth, making it easy to mistake him for a child half his age. And he'd long been living with the knowledge that his lungs were slowly but inevitably failing. By the day of his graduation, they were profoundly weakened, and he'd begun needing a steady flow of supplemental oxygen all the time. On that day, however, we were gathered for a joyful celebration. Eric's family was incredibly proud of him (I'll admit I was pretty proud too), and he was getting ready to go to college. The choices of the previous year had brought him to this moment, and this young man, all of eighteen years old, had blazed his own path to it.

Soon after our very first meeting, Eric used his developing hypnosis skills solely to help him breathe more easily. As he became more skilled, he began to use them to help him get to sleep. He used them to ease his anxiety over the decision we'd begun discussing not long after his sixteenth birthday: the choice about getting on the waiting list for a lung transplant. In time, he became one of the most gifted self-hypnotists I've worked with—able to utilize his skills to bring calm into his life and chase out pain at will. As he did so, his confidence steadily grew.

Realistically, a transplant was the only thing that could keep Eric alive once his weakening lungs failed, but contemplating undergoing such a radical procedure was a daunting, terrifying step for a teenager. Not only was the procedure itself scary to contemplate, but, following a transplant, the average patient lived for only five years. Thus a lung transplant fell far short of a cure. If the need for an organ transplant had arisen in a moment of emergency, like a car accident, the decision would have been made for him and likely without hesitation. But this was someone who had been living with disease all his life, who had adapted and persevered, and who could not possibly know what future date would be too late to choose such a drastic option. Eric had built a full life, making friends and going to school, running for a position as a class officer, planning for higher education, and being part of his close-knit family. It was no easy decision to step away from everything that made his daily life fulfilling to undergo a difficult and risky surgery that would change everything—especially while his lungs were still working, though in a diminished capacity.

When he was seventeen, Eric chose to visit the transplant center in a city 250 miles away and then made the complex decision to get on the waiting list. But shortly after his eighteenth birthday, when they told his family he was nearing the top of the list and should be awaiting a call regarding a lung transplant, his ambivalence reached its peak. He relied on hypnosis to calm and center himself, but the choice weighed on him. During one of our appointments, I helped him reframe the decision.

At that time it was unclear whether Eric's lung disease would stabilize or continue to deteriorate rapidly. "If you were able to live indefinitely the way you're feeling now," I asked, "would that be acceptable to you?"

His answer came quickly. "Yes," he said. "I'm doing pretty well."

Not long afterward, in the middle of his senior year of high school, donor lungs became available, and Eric chose to turn them down. The transplant program would give him one more chance, but there was no way to know when or whether that opportunity would come or if he'd be able to accept it. Either choice carried dire risk, but Eric had had a lot of time to think about what he would do, and he was quietly confident in his decision. His family and his doctors respected his choice.

Instead of taking the transplant, he finished and graduated high school, celebrated with his friends and family, spent much of a happy summer in his sunny backyard, moved into a dorm with all his breathing medicine and equipment, took classes, and made friends. He was living life fully and on his own terms.

Several months later, when Eric suffered a lung collapse, I rushed to the intensive care unit, where a team was preparing to put in a chest tube. He wanted to use hypnosis to ease the process, and even though he was capable of doing that on his own, in the unsettling energy of his room, I talked him through it, reminding him of his calming place and the healing light that shone on him there. His breathing eased, and in a few minutes the tube was placed.

Afterward, Eric thanked me for being with him and asked, earnestly, "Are you optimistic about me?"

"Yes," I said. "Always."

Eric occupied much of his time in the hospital by watching videos with his family and playing computer games. He loved jokes, so his mom would bring pages of them to giggle over together. On one occasion, Eric gave himself the hypnotic suggestion that he would find his name to be the funniest word he had ever heard. That day, when I said, "Eric," he burst out laughing. His cheeks dimpled and his eyes watered and he shook so hard I worried he'd further damage his lungs. I hated to do it, but I had to ask him to remove the suggestion so he wouldn't hurt himself. This, too, made him laugh, as he gently ribbed me for having shown him the tools to do it in the first place.

Eric told me he often did hypnosis while he was alone in the hospital, that even while he was attached to the chest tube, the practice made him feel like he could remove himself from the stress and pain of the place. When he was feeling well, he had lots of visitors, and he was always a favorite of the nurses. When one of them asked how he was maintaining such a positive attitude, he quipped, "When you're sick, it doesn't pay to be irritable—that's when you need your friends the most!"

When it became apparent that Eric's lung collapse was not going to heal well enough for him to go home from the hospital, he and his family decided it was time to get him to the transplant center before his lungs became so diseased that he could not be transferred safely. That day I thanked him for allowing me to be a part of his life and told him I'd always remember him. He told me he had no regrets about the choices he'd made, that he was glad he'd gotten to finish school and go to college.

As he was loaded into the ambulance that would transport him to the airport, Eric said, "I will always remember you," and waved good-bye. Over the three years I'd known him, I'd seen that Eric viewed the world in a positive light, just like I do. I prayed that light would help him.

Hypnosis didn't cure Eric's lung disease, but it enhanced his control over his life in novel ways that let him face his condition with confidence and competence. I was deeply proud of all he'd accomplished and the way this small young man had stood tall and claimed his life as his own.

WHAT YOU CAN DO ON YOUR OWN

A physician who prompts a patient to utilize the mind's abilities gains the benefit of a whole new tool set with which to help—one that is readily at the disposal of the child. Parents can also prompt children to use their own tools, to look inward rather than outward for solutions. Simple ways to begin fostering this mind-set at home include directly involving your child in discussions about their health, whether in your clinician's office or at home. If your child is frustrated with a treatment or a medication, ask what they think can be done to make it easier on them. If you have multiple options available to address a medical or behavioral issue, present them to your child in the form of choices—and then respect their preference and support their efforts.

Ultimately, we all want our children to be able to identify, assess, and deal with their own problems. We want them to ask for help when *they* need it rather than presuming that they need help all the time. It's never too soon to start fostering this attitude by treating children as equal partners in solving their problems.

18

Peace with the Past

The Beneficial Effects of Memory Reconstruction

There are countless ways the events of the past shape our present. They are like small construction blocks of who we are—what we've perceived with our senses, whom we've known, where we've been, and what we've done—all interlocking to help build the conscious and subconscious of each individual. Some of those blocks take up more space than others, among them foundational moments that help us define ourselves in both positive and negative ways. A child's memories of welcoming a sibling or winning an award or stargazing in the backyard with a parent, for example, might become significant positive forces to which they can return again and again. These powerful memories can serve as a touchstone to remind kids that they are part of a family, capable of excellence, or dearly loved and help them develop a strong sense of their own identities.

Almost inevitably, some of those big "blocks" of consciousness become occupied by negative associations—like times a child was injured or suffered a loss or felt afraid. These are normal parts of who we are, but for some children (and adults) those negative experiences become disproportionately present in their lives—they get hung up on them to the point of becoming distracted or frustrated or even exhibiting anxiety-based symptoms of illness. The offending block can even be a gap—a nagging sense that a memory of something important is missing. And some experts believe that at times that's exactly the case, because sometimes the subconscious represses an experience that is too painful to process or integrate into conscious awareness.[1]

Guided hypnosis can be a highly effective tool in helping patients work through events from the past that are causing them pain or dysfunction in the present. With the help of this tool, children can imagine revisiting past experiences in a way that feels safe and controlled, and they can change the ways they perceive those moments. This method can help them accept and move on from past traumas, put events that have been disproportionately disturbing into context, and overcome phobias based in memories of fear and anxiety.

We must bear in mind that not only can memories recovered in hypnosis be inaccurate, but some may not even have occurred. Sometimes the patient's subconscious makes memories up because a clinician has asked questions in a leading way. In fact, memory recall as a result of hypnosis can be so inaccurate that memories recovered during hypnosis are often not admissible as evidence in a court of law. From a therapeutic standpoint, however, a false memory can still serve as a useful metaphor that can help promote healing.

TAKING THE FEAR OUT OF PHOBIAS

My patient Chloe internalized another child's traumatic moment, and her case is a good representation of how hypnosis can recalibrate a child's fear by putting the original incident into new focus.

I met Chloe when she was eleven and her overwhelming and constant fear of throwing up was dominating many aspects of her life. She was exceedingly careful about what she ate. She was afraid to go to school because her mother would not be there to comfort her, if necessary, or to help her clean up if she vomited; she'd sometimes develop an actual stomachache because of her stress. She was afraid to travel in the car on long rides. And whenever she went to a new place, she felt compelled to immediately find the bathroom so she'd know where she could run if she felt like she was going to be sick.

Chloe's parents had done everything they could think of to alleviate this irrational fear (irrational because this child had only thrown up twice in her life—both times in the privacy of her home when she had the flu). Chloe's fear was based not in her own experience but in an incident she'd witnessed when she was seven years old in the second grade. At that time, one of her classmates had been sick in front of the entire class, had cried because she was embarrassed, and had afterward been teased and called a sissy by some of the other children.

During the incident, Chloe felt a mounting sense of anxiety and fear, so much so that her heart was pounding and she started to sweat and feel a little sick herself. Afterward she developed her own intense fear of throwing up, one that was getting worse instead of easing as time passed.

I taught Chloe how to use hypnosis and calm herself with a relaxation sign (crossing her fingers). Once she'd mastered the basic techniques, I asked whether I could help her overcome her fear by teaching her to use ideomotor signaling. She very much hoped to put this fear behind her, so she wanted to learn.

Once Chloe mastered the basics of allowing her subconscious to lift one finger for *No*, another for *Yes*, and a third for *I don't want to say*, I began a dialogue with it, asking, "Would you be willing to help Chloe with her fear of throwing up?"

She raised her pointer finger. *Yes.*

"Great," I said. "Please go back in your mind to the day Chloe first developed this fear, when she was in second grade. Let me know when you get there."

The *Yes* finger rose again.

"Now," I continued, "please teach young Chloe how to calm herself with her relaxation sign. Let me know when you've done that."

Yes.

"Great. Now, please have young Chloe reexperience the day when her friend threw up. This time, when it happens, she will cross her fingers, and she can remain calm. Let me know when this has been done."

Yes.

"Great. Did you notice how Chloe never developed any fear that day because she was calm?"

Yes.

"Is Chloe still afraid of throwing up?"

No.

Out of hypnosis, Chloe confirmed that her memory of what happened that day had changed, that she felt sorry her classmate had been sick but knew she was OK throughout the incident and after.

If Chloe had experienced multiple disturbing events of throwing up in her past, we would likely have moved on to each of those, allowing her subconscious to remind her to remain calm. Her case, though, was traceable back to a single bad day, and her disruptive fear was banished by helping her alter how she remembered feeling on that one occasion.

In some ways, especially when the problem is a phobia, this kind of intervention is among the most straightforward and effective uses of hypnosis. When a patient revisits the scene where an irrational fear developed and changes how they feel about it, their anxiety tends to resolve quickly. My patients have used this technique to put to rest all kinds of phobias—fears of everything from spiders, snakes, and bees to dogs and clowns, to flying and driving, to needles and dentists, to, of course, the awfulness of developing an illness or throwing up.

TONING DOWN A MEMORY

In many ways, memory is in the realm of the subconscious, where most of what we know from the past can be reasonably considered to have been constructed by the subconscious mind. We can recognize this anytime we think of a past event and picture ourselves in it. Since we were never standing outside ourselves looking on, we know that somehow the mind has created a mental snapshot of the moment.

Working to plumb the depths of a child's memory is careful work—especially because it is a sad truth that not all problems rooted in our pasts are as easily resolved as simple phobias. The process of helping children make peace with past memories involves guiding them to achieve a sense of control over their fears and stresses as they work through them. An effective method that I use frequently for this purpose involves helping patients view memories on an imagined movie screen where they can change their perception by controlling the film. For example, the child can stop and start the movie, turn down its sound, or switch it to black and white. Each means of managing the way they perceive the memory is not only a way to make it easier to review but also a metaphor for taking control of its content.

Importantly, the more difficulty a child is having with their past and the more traumatic the event, the more critical it is to create distance between the child and their memories. In many cases, I enlist the help of the subconscious in this process, asking whether the patient is ready to handle the emotions that may come rushing in as they work through a difficult memory. If the subconscious says the child isn't ready, then the subconscious can be invited to recall the memory instead of suggesting that the child do so consciously—creating yet another layer of protection for the child's emotions. The crux of the technique—creating a "this is your life" experience—relies on the clinician respecting whatever level of distance the child needs, from a metaphorical front-row seat to a position standing just outside the door, only beginning to consciously think about what's happening in the room.

Going back to an original trauma, sometimes termed age regression, is often best done in slow, methodical steps that narrow the distance between the present and the traumatic past event, letting kids learn one step at a time how to teach the younger version of themselves the tools they've learned to calm themselves. With each step, the child can gently overwrite the memory—not necessarily the events that occurred but the way the child experienced them. Researchers have found that patients given a medication that calms them (propranolol) during a traumatic event are less likely to develop posttraumatic stress disorder.[2] I have wondered whether children who are coached to remain calm in hypnosis as they imagine a traumatic event achieve a similar benefit in prevention or resolution of long-term psychological problems. Throughout this process, I'm able to remind patients that they've come through well, that they've moved past the moments of trauma that hurt them. I ask many of them to tell their younger selves that they are going to survive and be OK, that their future selves are strong and resilient and equipped with the tools they need to move on from things that happened in the past.

Another, related version of this kind of hypnosis involves projection into the future through age progression. Children are invited to imagine a future in which their problem has resolved and to describe in detail what life will be like without it. Then I ask how they get from where they are to where they want to be. We talk about the steps they can take and which should be first. Envisioning a future in which they're doing better gives kids a reason and confidence to continue using their hypnosis and to take progressive steps in the direction they want to go.

It is important to note that some memories are best left undisturbed. Clinicians and parents can make logical and protective cases for how and when to consider this possibility, but I've found that each child's subconscious is usually the best authority on what a child can and cannot handle. If the adults involved are unsure, using hypnosis to ask the subconscious for guidance may be a critical step in ensuring a child's care doesn't put too great of an emotional strain on the patient.

A GAP IN TIME

Early in the days when I was learning to guide patients in hypnosis, Paul had a few vague memories of a childhood hospitalization and near-death experience when he was seven years old that had continued to haunt him into his late teens. At the time, Paul had been placed on a ventilator for the first time, and even though he and his family rarely spoke about the incident, when they did, it was reverently, conveying the distinct sense that this had been a traumatic time for all of them.

Paul was keen to better understand what had happened. Even after we obtained the hospital records and I explained everything I could glean from them, he still had unanswered questions and only disquietingly nonspecific memories of what had occurred.

I offered to help Paul try to revisit this time, to guide his hypnosis to access his subconscious memories. Remarkably, as he reviewed the day, more than a decade in the past, Paul seemed to remember every detail. He remembered being in the hospital for an asthma attack, feeling better, and thinking he'd be going home soon. He remembered being served the chicken soup that was later discovered to have contained a milk by-product. He saw himself eating it and feeling his throat constrict. He saw the doctors who rushed in and panicked at his bedside, and he remembered one of them ushering his mother out of the room. He felt the pain and pressure of the breathing tube being placed while he was still alert and awake (because there was no time to sedate him), and he remembered how it felt to be whisked down the hall, out into the open air, and onto the waiting helicopter that would take him to a bigger medical center. Paul remembered that the foremost thought in his mind as he was rushed through this process was his worry that his mom would not be able to be with him.

At the end of his hypnosis session that morning, Paul was thoughtful and confident.

"I finally understand," he said. "I've always needed to know what happened to me that day. Now I do."

As he left the office, I realized that even if Paul's recollection was not accurate, it had allowed him to come to terms with a traumatic event that had been bothering him for most of his life.

I couldn't have known that we would not have long—less than a year—before a catastrophic allergic reaction to a milk product at college would claim Paul, leaving everyone who loved him struggling to find peace after losing a young man who was a bright light in each of our lives.

WHAT YOU CAN DO ON YOUR OWN

Hypnosis can be a highly effective way of helping children move from an immersed perspective of a negative past event to one that helps them view and deal with it from what feels like a safe distance. It is not, however, the only way, and any child can benefit from practicing simple techniques to put their hardships into a larger and more comprehensive context. You can facilitate this with your child in a number of ways, starting with demonstrating by your own example that some things are not worth getting or staying upset about. For example, if you lose or break something, focus on what happens next rather than what's already happened. If you suffer a setback at work or at home, show your child that what matters even more than the negative event is how you are going to respond to it. And when your child makes a mistake, help them focus on how they can correct it or move forward rather than on the damage that's occurred.

When your child is struggling to come to terms with difficult events, encourage them to try to take a more distant view, to take themselves out of the moment. For young children, you can suggest another impartial observer to assess the situation to help them shift perspective (one study found simply asking kids "What would Batman do?" helped them better use reason over emotion to make decisions).[3] Asking what an impartial observer would think can give them a little room to feel less caught up in the moment (live or in memory) and a little more circumspect.

Just as we can use shifts of time in hypnosis to help kids cope with hardships, you can do the same at home, asking your child if a troubling event will matter in a week or a month or a year. Looking ahead can offer hope that something that seems big and scary today will one day seem small and forgettable in the rearview mirror.

Lastly, even though it's important to acknowledge your child's pain in troubled times, it's also possible to offer a glimpse of an upside of most things and thus reconstruct how the child perceives a situation: throwing up is the body's way of protecting itself; an accident without an injury is a near miss (rather than a catastrophe); or a failed test can provide an impetus to learn a new, better study skill.

The Grieving Child

Pathways to Catharsis

Human life is a balance of dark and light, and none of us—even children—is immune to the darkness of death and loss. Grappling with the first or a profound loss in childhood can be especially tough on kids because they haven't yet developed the coping tools to help them process and accept dramatic shifts in their lives. Their limited experience offers them a narrow perspective, and many find it difficult to believe that tragedy is part of life or that they can and will be able to feel happy or hopeful again. In a gentle world, children would be introduced to the idea of loss gradually, giving them the opportunity to learn how to respond and deal with their feelings. But, of course, the world is not always gentle, and sometimes hard emotional challenges come to children who are ill prepared to face them.[1]

Not surprisingly, many things can bring a child to great grief besides the death of a loved one, among them the loss of a pet, the loss of a two-parent home after a divorce, or the loss of a close friend because of a falling out or even a move. Many also, in their own ways, grieve the end of childhood and their loss of innocence. A small minority, like Jared, my patient with cystic fibrosis, and Eric, my patient on the lung transplant list, thread their way through the uniquely challenging grief of knowing their own lives will likely be short. Every day brings not just a theoretical possibility of death but the reality of its being near and coming closer.

Many times, I've treated children who come to the office because of physical or psychological symptoms that do not, on the surface, seem to have anything to do with grief. It can take time and trust for that cause to reveal itself. Hypnosis can serve as an equally effective tool both in figuring out what is causing a child's distress and in helping them find comfort and closure after loss. One of its unique benefits is in allowing children to use hypnotic imagery to have cathartic interactions and conversations with the person or pet or even an earlier version of themselves that they're missing. Many of them are able to use this tool to begin to mend and feel better.

A HEARTSICK BOY

My patient Charlie had suffered great loss in his twelve years. He'd lost both parents, his grandfather, his cat, and his home. He was angry and grieving, especially for his mother, who'd died just four months before we met. His uncle, with whom he was living, initially brought him to see me because his asthma was interfering with his sleep, but it quickly became clear that this was a child with a heavy heart who was dealing with much more than trouble using his inhaler.

I taught Charlie how to use hypnosis to calm himself. He imagined going to a waterfall in a forest, and he learned to associate making an OK sign with his left hand with the feeling of relaxation he achieved there. I encouraged him to practice and use this skill when he started feeling short of breath. He reported both that it helped him breathe more easily and that he was getting to sleep earlier and resting more soundly with the help of hypnosis.

It was obvious, though, that Charlie was struggling with and distraught over his mother's death. He was angry and unhappy most of the time. When we talked about what he'd been through, he told me he'd cried for his grandfather and his cat but not for his mom. He'd felt "like a stone" from the time of her funeral. Even though he'd already seen a counselor to help him deal with his feelings, he still felt cold to her and angry that she'd left him.

When I asked whether he could tell me why he was angry, Charlie explained, in heartbreaking detail, how even though he'd needed his mom to be healthy and stay with him, she wouldn't take care of herself. In the end, she'd died of complications of diabetes and liver disease while she was still a young woman.

When we spoke further about her, Charlie acknowledged that he knew his mother loved him and that she'd been a good person. But he still didn't think he could forgive her for abandoning him. "She should be here," he said. "She should be here right now."

Of course he was right. No child should have to lose a mother, and Charlie's loss was especially bitter because he didn't have another parent to lean on. He felt alone and frustrated. I was certain that until he found a way to deal with his anger and sadness, he would continue to suffer and be unable to accept her death. Like adults, children typically experience grief in stages, among them denial, anger, depression, and acceptance. The process is not necessarily linear, but whatever path would take Charlie to eventual acceptance, it was clear during our appointments that he was mired in the quicksand of negative emotions and not moving forward. Sometimes in traditional talk therapy, counselors role-play critical conversations their patients need to have to help them deal with their feelings. In this case, I thought Charlie needed the chance to have a missed conversation with his mother and hopefully to be reminded of her loving presence. Rather than act the part, I suggested an option that's only available in the unique therapy we were doing together.

"Charlie," I said, "would you be interested in talking with your mother in hypnosis?"

"Yes," he said, cocking his head. "Can you do that?"

"I can't, but you can if you want to. You can go into hypnosis, next to your waterfall, and invite your mother to join you. I believe she will come. Once she arrives, you can imagine spending as much time as you like with her and talking with her. When you're done, you can come back."

Charlie closed his eyes, inhaled deeply, and settled back in his seat. He was quiet for a few minutes and then opened his eyes, wide and wet with tears.

"I saw her," he whispered.

"What did she say?"

"She said she loves me."

"What did you say?"

"I love her."

"Anything else?" I asked.

"We sat together," he said. "She held my hand."

"And how do you feel?"

"I feel a lot better," he said, exhaling heavily.

And then he smiled and added, "I told her I forgive her."

I told Charlie it would be OK to visit his mother in hypnosis anytime he needed her, that she wanted to help him feel at peace. This was a first step in relieving the anger that had been seething inside him since her death.

When I asked him how real the interaction had seemed, Charlie confidently replied, "It *was* real."

"Do you believe you actually saw your mom?"

"Yes," he said. "I did."

"I think you may be right," I said, going along with my patient. "If you are open to seeing souls, I believe you can see them using hypnosis."

He nodded.

"In fact, I have heard that young kids can see souls more easily than adults."

"My cousin is two," he said, "and he talks to my mom all the time."

"I'm not surprised," I responded. "Some people think many toddlers can see souls or spirits. No one has taught them that they're not supposed to perceive them yet."

I have treated many other patients who reported with absolute certainty that while in hypnosis they'd communicated with the ghost or soul of a relative. I couldn't know if Charlie had or had not met his mother's soul, but I did know that he needed to have the conversation he'd had with her and that he needed me to believe his reporting of it, to validate his experience. When both of those things had happened, he became able to move past his consuming grief and into the next phase of his life.

Interacting with an imagined loved one is often cathartic, whether the loved one is alive or dead. Just as a patient can experience an interaction that helps settle grief, they can also use this tool to resolve other feelings. For example, a child can be taught and encouraged to direct loving, kind thoughts toward a family member, teacher, or friend. Thinking things like *May you be happy, may you be healthy, may you be at peace* is sometimes the first step in mending relationships the child perceives as stressful or painful. The improvement could be the result of a child's change in attitude, but some children also believe their thoughts influence those of the chosen individual.

A FRIEND IN COMMON

Children often inadvertently use symptoms to resolve problems when they don't have better ways to cope. This was the case for Serena, who came to see me about her severe migraine headaches. Serena had suffered headaches since she was small, but when she was twelve years old, they reached the point of being debilitating. She was in so much pain and getting so little relief from medications that her pediatrician referred her for a neurological workup. After consultations and numerous tests, including a brain scan, the neurologist found no discernible cause for Serena's pain. As a last resort, he referred her to me.

At my office in the medical center, Serena told me that she was having headaches every day and that they typically lasted for several hours. It had been a year since the headaches had gotten this bad, and she felt that nothing really helped ease them once they started. Naps, medications, heating pads, ice, meditation—none of it was working. Her father reported that she was missing school, losing sleep, and not eating healthfully.

When I started to tell Serena about hypnosis and how it might help her, she politely interrupted and told me she knew a lot about it already, because her good friend and neighbor Paulie had used it all the time. I have to believe it was some unique intention or balance of the universe that brought Serena to me, because her friend Paulie was my beloved patient Paul—the young man who'd inspired me to make hypnosis a central part of my practice of medicine. The discovery of our mutual friend immediately bonded me to Serena and her family, especially when I learned how close they'd been. She described Paul as "like a brother," and her father characterized him as the son he'd never had. Paul's death had plunged all the members of Serena's family into grief, and in the year since his passing, they'd struggled to find ways to talk about their feelings about it, even among themselves. Each of them carried a private and intense sense of loss.

For Serena, the youngest and therefore least equipped of the family to deal with these feelings, I began to suspect her intensified headaches were an expression of the anger, sorrow, and frustration she felt about losing her friend. She and her father had both placed the onset of the terrible headaches at about a year prior to our first meeting, which would have been soon after Paul's death.

I told Serena I thought hypnosis might be helpful for her, as migraines are known to resolve with its regular use.[2] I also thought I might be able to help her with her grief over Paul, especially as we both knew him well.

She proved to be a good pupil, quickly learning to use hypnosis to relax. I encouraged her to use it for this purpose every day, to reduce her tension. Because I thought her symptoms might be associated with Paul's death, I felt it was important to explore the possibility. To do so, I suggested that Serena imagine herself having a headache. Once she did so, I suggested she remove the headache from her body and let it stand next to her.

"I am not sure what your headache will look like," I said. "Perhaps it will look like a person, a creature, or a thing. But you will recognize it. Once you see it, you can ask it why it has been causing you pain."

Serena reported that her headache appeared to be a girl named Mary, who looked just like her. Mary explained that she was causing Serena headaches because she had not dealt with Paulie's death. I suggested Serena ask Mary what kind of deal she could make in return for stopping the headaches. Mary told her that as long as Serena would begin dealing with losing her friend so she could get on with her life, she'd stop the headaches.

Serena agreed to this plan.

At the end of her hypnosis session, she said she felt better and that she wanted to discuss Paul's death. We discussed how Serena missed his physical presence and his supportiveness. It is an unusual circumstance for a doctor to be mourning the same person as the patient, but even though I had made my own peace with Paul's passing, I found myself also missing his presence and remembering how his active and curious mind had challenged and inspired me.

I asked Serena what she thought Paul would have wanted her to do at this time, and she said he'd tell her to make new friends and be more confident. Serena seemed visibly relieved that she was able to talk to someone about Paul's death. She said she'd done very little of that over the past year.

Three weeks later Serena reported that she'd had just one headache since I'd seen her last. When I complimented her on using hypnosis so well, I asked about her routine with it. She said she'd been practicing it every afternoon to relax.

Then she added shyly, "Sometimes I've seen Paulie."

Wow. This was not something I'd suggested. It seemed that Serena was moving ahead in her grieving process largely on her own. Being able to imagine talking to Paul was a positive therapeutic step.

"Where did you see him?" I asked.

"In my relaxing place."

"And did you talk?"

She nodded. "He told me that he's fine. He said he wanted me to make new friends and that he could talk to me whenever I wanted."

"That's wonderful," I said. "It seems you've found a way to keep him alive in your mind. I know you've missed his support. I'm glad you can have that again when you think about him and talk to him."

Serena rarely had headaches over the next several months. When I discharged her from my care, I sent up a silent thanks to our mutual friend. Wherever he was and whatever connection he still had with the people he cared about, the indelible mark he'd made in our lives was still warm and positive. I was certain that somewhere in the universe his spirit remained very much alive.

WHAT YOU CAN DO ON YOUR OWN

Sometimes children experience anticipatory grief: they know a loss is coming, and they're already in mourning. You may not be able to change the circumstances of the situation your child is grieving, but you can take steps to help them make choices in the present that will ultimately help them cope. If your child has a sick relative, for example, ask whether there's something they'd like to say to or do for that person. They might choose to give flowers or share a favorite book or write a letter. If a family pet is ill, give kids the opportunity to do something that makes the animal happy. I know a family who baked doggie cookies and another who had a "Rufus Day" in which they thought of all the things that might make the dog happy—like cuddling on the couch or playing on a picnic blanket in the sun—and did them.

After a death, you can still help your child feel better by encouraging them to send good wishes to their loved one and to know it's OK to continue to communicate with them in their own way. I have a patient who tells me he talks with the spirit of his old dog all the time, which always makes him feel better. Another received a notebook after the death of her beloved grandmother, and she writes her letters in it, telling her what's going on in her own life and asking what's happening in heaven. Children can plant memorial flowers and trees, or they can participate in an activity that was special to the person they lost.

All these steps will help your child create positive memories. In many ways, memories are the bridge we all share between the present and the past, the living and the dead. If your child is lucky enough to have time to make a few more good memories before a loss, then those will help them deal with their grief in the long term. Even after a loss has already happened, opening a dialogue about memories is often a good first step to healing and acceptance.

Finding Spirituality Within

Strength Gained from New Perspectives

The delicate privilege of dealing, sometimes directly, with the subconscious minds of children has often given me a unique insight into the inner workings of their spirituality. They are of diverse conscious faiths; they are practicing and nonpracticing Christians, Jews, Muslims, and Buddhists, followers of other religions, and adherents of no formal religion at all. Some have been raised in homes where faith plays a central role in their upbringing; many, in homes where it plays little to none. The concept of spirituality in patient care is broad, encompassing a feeling of being part of something larger than the self. In the context of organized religious institutions, it's the feeling of being part of a world created and loved by a higher power. In nature, it may be feeling part of a great and beautiful universe. In the arts, it might come in the form of a transcendent moment, experiencing a creation that seems to prove the existence of perfect inspiration in an imperfect world.

Spirituality often entails a relationship with something existing outside the five senses, and it can encompass faith in God or perceived connection with another guiding entity. Alternatively, a spiritual state can develop through communication with one's wiser and older subconscious. Even a thoughtful examination of perspective can open up our spiritual side when we choose to view the human condition in terms of our entire lives or even generations—a vantage point from which we can consider individual life events as parts of a greater whole. In almost any form, spirituality helps children gain perspective on their difficulties and encourages resilience. A spiritual perspective helps them navigate challenges more effectively because it gives them a sense of purpose in their lives. Without a spiritual sense, when times are hard, a child can easily think, *I have bad luck* or *I got dealt the wrong cards.* With a spiritual understanding, the same child can think, *I have this challenge and there is a reason for it* or *This is not random; it's supposed to strengthen me.* This shift of mind-set is empowering. It can help children weather difficulties and actively engage in overcoming them. It can endow them with the will and strength to build new or better relationships, to do better in school or sports, and to engage in service to others (something they almost universally want to do but often don't know how). Having a sense of purpose can serve as a foundation for both physical and mental health, and I see this every day in the outcomes of my patients.

Encouraging a child's spiritual side can equally help them cope with hardships that are outside their realm of influence. An eleven-year-old patient was referred to me for shortness of breath, and it quickly became apparent that her symptom was rooted in anxiety, as it never occurred at night or when she was engaged in a distracting activity. The girl's mother had been diagnosed with cancer and was undergoing a chemotherapy regimen that was making her sick. The girl understandably felt powerless to help her mom. When we talked about what she believed in, she told me she had faith in God and knew God heard her prayers. We talked about how she could help her mother by praying for her, and even this small shift from inaction to action helped relieve her respiratory symptoms.

I believe the human psyche is constructed in a way that yearns for growth and increased health. Given a path to achieving this through spirituality, children are generally curious and enthusiastic to learn.

One of these paths is through hypnosis. In many ways, it is a state similar to those evoked by prayer or experiencing awe-inspiring nature or art. In each, children feel open to connecting to something beyond themselves. Teaching children about the existence of their subconscious and how to interact with it helps them develop their spiritual side—in whatever form that takes.

WHAT WOULD YOU CHANGE TODAY?

Versions of the serenity prayer—asking for strength not only to make changes but also to know when to accept things as they are—go back at least to ancient Greece. The Stoic philosopher Epictetus wrote, "Make the best use of what is in your power, and take the rest as it happens."

To help children with chronic illness develop perspective, I sometimes ask them, "Suppose you had the opportunity to trade in your disease for good health. But in exchange, you would have to give up everything you've gained from your illness, such as your appreciation of the extent of your family's love for you, the friends you met as the result of your disease, and the wisdom you've gained from your experiences. Would you make the trade?"

Surprisingly, most children answer no, including those who are in the process of dying. Once children reflect upon their answer, they often develop the empowering realization that they are able to embrace their illness and thus be more at peace with it.

This kind of acceptance of what is can be freeing for kids. For example, I had a fourteen-year-old patient named Drew who was born many weeks early and had experienced a number of health issues related to his prematurity. He'd developed a speech impediment I suspected was caused by a psychological issue rather than a "hard-wired" neurological problem, because at times he was quite eloquent. In addition, he was unhappy and overly self-conscious much of the time, and he'd developed some behavioral tics like constant sniffling, which suggested he was feeling anxious.[1]

After I taught Drew to use hypnosis and ideomotor signaling, he was willing and able to let his subconscious speak with me directly. During our conversation, I asked how Drew was feeling.

"He's sad," Drew's subconscious answered.

When I probed as to why, it answered that Drew had many difficulties related to his prematurity. One of these was that his peers frequently made fun of him because he was small.

"Has Drew gained anything by having been born prematurely?" I asked.

"Yes."

"What has he gained?"

"He likes himself," the subconscious answered. "He has a kind, self-reliant personality because of learning how to deal with his medical difficulties."

"Is there anything else?" I asked.

"There are some advantages to being small," he said. "He can do things other people can't, like climbing into small spaces or running under people when he plays basketball." He thought a bit more and then said, "I think he's happy now that he was born premature."

I suggested that Drew's subconscious should share these things with him and remind him that he was a resilient, smart, kind person.

Out of hypnosis, Drew didn't recall any of the conversation I'd had with his subconscious, and he agreed to continue practicing hypnosis to calm himself and overcome his speech difficulties.

The following week, Drew showed up for his appointment walking tall. He had not hesitated in his speech since I'd seen him last, and his mother noted that he'd also stopped sniffling all the time. When I congratulated him on his success and asked how he was feeling about this, Drew unzipped his sweat jacket and pointed to the grey T-shirt underneath. There, emblazoned in bright blue letters, it said, "I Have Decided to Put Myself in Charge."

Accessing his subconscious allowed Drew to gain a spiritual perspective on his life, one that was transformative. I went home smiling that day, wishing the same kind of self-guided success Drew had accomplished for each of my patients.

NOURISHING THE SPIRIT

I had the privilege of working with a seventeen-year-old patient who was going through a crushing confluence of difficulties—among them living with an alcoholic parent, struggling with depression, and making an unfortunate, avoidable mistake that put him in the legal system. Nonetheless, he was doing well in school and actively planning for a career. This was a good person who had made some poor choices (like almost all children and adolescents do) and had some troubling circumstances pushed upon him. He had a strong spirit, and I hoped to reach that spirit when I told him at our first meeting, "You are an amazing person. Despite all of your difficulties, you are doing so well. Obviously, you are very important to this world."

Another patient with depression told me that he started feeling much better about himself after we met for the first time.

I had asked, "If you had only one wish, what would it be?"

He raised his eyes to the ceiling as he pondered the question. "I think I wouldn't want to make the wish now. I'd save it for when I really need it."

"That's a great answer," I exclaimed. "I've never heard anyone else answer that way."

Years later, the patient told me that this simple exchange had made him realize he was special and could contribute to the world. This patient now is thinking of a career as a counselor.

Each of these young patients benefited from an honest reminder of a simple fact: every person is a unique and special soul, and each of us has something valuable to contribute. Kids going through difficult times need to hear this. I believe that parents, teachers, and clinicians can better help the children in their care by taking a moment from time to time to reset conversations with reminders that the child is special, loved, and important. Kind words, shared with honest intentions, nourish the spirit.

SELF-UNDERSTANDING

As they mature, many teenagers grapple with questions regarding the meaning of their lives. This is especially true of children who live with chronic health problems, but it can lead any child to the development of anxiety or depression. Exploring the existential questions that bother them with the help of their subconscious has yielded some fascinating answers. Some of these include that the purpose of life is different for each individual and that it is up to each person to define their own meaning. Some have said the purpose of life is to help each other. Others have suggested that different people use different tools to make their mark on the world, like the written word, music, art, acting, counseling, healing, building, or donating.

One patient with a particularly complex and challenging medical history who practiced hypnosis for years spent only one session in all that time allowing his subconscious to write. The result of that session was a simple but powerful three-word statement: *Believe in me.* When I asked this very special young man what he thought it meant, he indicated it was an obvious admonition for him to be more confident in himself—a reassuring *You got this* from within.

In my practice, I give patients wrist bands that state, "Remember who you are," as a reminder of their source of wisdom within. Sometimes when children are feeling low, when they're struggling to find meaning, gentle reinforcement of their positive identity can help them recenter themselves. Over the years I've been amazed at how many patients develop a more spiritual outlook on their own circumstances and those of others once they discover the subconscious as a source of inner sagacity. It inspires them to believe in themselves and to look at the world with a little more wisdom and understanding. It is impossible to quantify the value of this change in outlook, but I've never seen it do anything but strengthen and encourage the children who achieve it.

WHAT YOU CAN DO ON YOUR OWN

As a parent, you can encourage your child to recognize the power and beauty of the spiritual world. The obvious suggestion is to make a habit of practicing whatever religion gives you and your family a spiritual home. Going to a house of worship reminds us of our spiritual power. Spirituality, though, goes beyond the bounds of any religion, and children should be encouraged to seek, recognize, and embrace things that help them appreciate the world's beauty and their place in it.

- Get out into nature. The naturalist John Muir wrote, "The clearest way into the universe is through a forest wilderness," and for as long as people have been walking the earth, it's true that we've been inspired by its beauty and felt closer to our spiritual selves in nature. Every child can benefit from getting outside.[2]
- Find an awesome place to visit—in person if you can or even on the web. One of my patients recently discovered, while she was recovering from surgery, that she could choose to view hours of footage from some of the most beautiful places in the world on her streaming service instead of constantly trying to find a television show.
- Listen to inspiring music. Music is a powerful tool in medicine, and countless studies show how it can support healing and wellness.[3] What inspires differs from person to person, but to encourage your child to get in touch with their inner spirituality, suggest they listen to music without lyrics so they can fill in their own meaning. The music of any formal religion in which you participate also has unique spiritual power, imbued by the ritual of ceremony, shared experience, and, in many cases, years or even centuries of tradition.
- Do something for another person. There may be no faster shortcut to a sense of being part of something larger than ourselves than doing good works. Your child can do something as simple as saying a prayer for a loved one or baking cookies for a neighbor or as involved as organizing trash collection at a park, building a mini library, or volunteering at a tutoring center for kids needing homework help.[4]

21

Ripples from the Center

How Hypnosis Helps Families Function

Any intervention that helps patients helps entire families. After two decades of practicing hypnosis therapy, seeing families heal and move forward continues to deepen my commitment to making this treatment more widely available. Parents often torment themselves over their children's health problems, and most will go to any lengths to help. Siblings respond in many ways. Some work especially hard to be self-sufficient so they don't draw resources their brother or sister needs, sometimes leaning in to demonstrate their willingness to help and sometimes distancing themselves as they try to establish identities separate from the person in their family who tends to require the most time and attention. Like children with chronic mental and physical health issues, families can and often do grow and become more empathetic and resilient as they deal with these challenges. But they can also feel beaten down by them and at a loss—especially when they can't find ways to help their loved one.[1]

Because hypnosis is a tool that puts the patient in the driver's seat, I've been blessed to witness countless families become stronger and happier as their children learned to manage their own symptoms, to feel better, and to carry themselves with greater confidence. One patient who comes to mind whenever I think of the potential for hypnosis is Larry, a young teen with cystic fibrosis, needle phobia, and illness-related anxiety who was my patient for many years. Larry was unforgettable as a person, in part because of his thoughtful nature and great love of history, and also because of his unique hypnosis experience.[2] With all the world, real and imagined, to choose from, Larry selected Theodore Roosevelt's Long Island home, circa the early 1900s, as his relaxing place. What's more, Larry reported having spoken with Roosevelt himself on occasion during hypnosis and said Roosevelt gave him guidance regarding how to feel better. Whether the Roosevelt of Larry's experience was a creation of his imagination, served as a metaphor, or represented an inner advisor from his subconscious (or some combination of the three), the interactions with him were instrumental in guiding Larry to a healthier, happier life. Following his Roosevelt and hypnotic relaxation experiences, Larry gained confidence and self-regulation skills that supported him in overcoming his insomnia, eliminating his chronic headaches, participating more at school, and even trying out for (and making) a sports team. Larry's health issues caused directly by his cystic fibrosis could not be resolved with hypnosis, but many other aspects of his day-to-day life improved because of it.

As is the case with all children dealing with health challenges, Larry's struggles impacted a circle of people outside himself. He lived with his parents and brother. He was loved by grandmothers, aunts, uncles, and cousins and deeply cared about by teachers, classmates, and teammates. When Larry was having a hard time, the people close to him, especially his family at home, shared that burden.

Over the first months Larry was using hypnosis, his behavior changed markedly. He stopped looking at the floor and started looking at me when we spoke. He smiled more quickly. He became eager to engage in conversations about topics that interested him. With many of his problematic symptoms managed, his performance in school improved—and with it his confidence.

During that time, it was impossible not to notice that Larry's mother's attitude was also changing. She'd initially come to the medical center visibly carrying the burden of her concern and caution in her slumped posture and reticence to engage. She'd been extremely quiet and shy, not wanting to ask for anything. She'd avoided making eye contact and kept to the corners of the room.

With each passing month, the changes in the way this loving parent carried herself seemed to reflect the changes Larry was experiencing. She began asking questions, making small talk, and shaking hands. She stood taller, spoke more clearly, and met my eyes when we carried on conversations.

After one memorable appointment when the three of us laughed out loud at a joke and then praised Larry's progress, I asked about this change, saying, "I think you've become more confident over the past few months. Do you?"

She looked a little surprised but nodded in the affirmative. "I do," she said. "I guess when Larry started feeling better, I started to feel better, too."

Larry continued to use hypnosis for years to deal with physical discomforts related to his cystic fibrosis and its therapies, to get enough sleep, to do better on tests, and to remain confident. By the time he was twenty-one and aged out of my care, he was on his way to a career as a translator and tutor, a smart, engaging young man with a positive outlook on the future. His family, too, was doing well. Even though they didn't directly participate in hypnosis, I have no doubt it was of benefit to them.

When one member of a family begins to heal, it can spark a self-propelling cycle of positivity: the child feels better, which makes the family feel better, which helps the child experience further improvement.

It's worth noting that even though Larry's mom didn't directly participate in hypnosis, many parents of children who learn this skill become adept at using it themselves. Sometimes parents start working on their own hypnosis abilities after sitting in on a child's instruction sessions, and others work with therapists of their own. There is certainly no age limit for who can benefit from this process.

PRECIOUS TIME

Nick, another a patient with cystic fibrosis, was in my care for much of his childhood. As for many children with severe and chronic pulmonary diseases, the deterioration of his lungs meant that one day the only hope for his life to go on would be a lung transplant. Nick's lungs failed more rapidly than those of most children with cystic fibrosis at that time. At the age of ten, he was already on a transplant waiting list, and his ability to function was impaired to the extent that he had to be homeschooled. He was spending hours of each day engaged in treatments to help keep his lungs clearer and functioning, and his medications consisted of an exhaustive regimen of nebulized, oral, and intravenous prescriptions.[3]

Nick learned to use hypnosis to calm and center himself, but as thirteen months passed in a holding pattern on the transplant list, he became frustrated and began to lose hope. First, he told his family that he wanted to stop doing his uncomfortable breathing therapy, then that he didn't want to stay on the transplant list, and finally that he believed in God and heaven and knew that if he died, he would be OK. He asked his family to help him make videos for his two preschool-aged sisters so that they could remember him.

Nick's parents and his entire medical team recognized the need to respect this child's preference not to continue to suffer each day, but we were loath to give up. I began wondering if there were any way to shift Nick's perspective to a more hopeful one without making false promises. During his next appointment, I asked him if he would accept a transplant if it were available that day, and he said he would.

"Perhaps you're not quite ready to give up fighting if you'd have the surgery today," I suggested. I asked if there were any changes we could make on that day that might help him, but aside from an adjustment to an uncomfortable airway-clearing therapy, he couldn't think of anything.

"There's nothing to look forward to," he said. "And there are no lungs for me."

"What do you wish you could be doing during this time, Nick?" I asked, employing the subtlest suggestion of possibility.

At this, he turned wistful, quietly saying, "I'd like to go crab fishing, on the Atlantic seaboard."

It seemed that he'd given this question some thought. It was also clear he believed this activity to be outside the realm of possibility.

When I said, "I think that's an excellent goal," he looked glum, maybe thinking I was patronizing him.

"Tell me what it would be like," I continued. "What do you think you would see and hear and smell there?"

Nick described cool, salty water, seagulls flying overhead, and a boat rocking in the waves with buoys hanging over its side and a pilothouse with windows. As he did so, he became increasingly animated and enthusiastic.

"That sounds wonderful," I said. "Let's see if there's any way to make it happen."

There was a way. Within twenty-four hours plans were in place for Nick and his family to travel 250 miles to the Jersey shore. Even after a multiday hospitalization two weeks later—just a week before his trip—it was clear to everyone involved that following through on the promise of the trip was necessary.

Before Nick left the hospital, we spoke about how there might be other things he'd like to plan and do after his trip to the shore, like maybe host a party for some of his friends. We had reached a point at which, with every word I uttered to this boy, I strove to convey just a little bit more hope, to share the possibility of a future. It was the subtlest form of hypnosis, using the power of words to create a positive, promising image of a day in the future.

Six days after his discharge from the hospital, while he was vacationing with his family at the shore, lungs became available for Nick. His initial response to hearing the long-awaited news was a surprising one: he said he didn't want to cut his trip short! At that moment I felt quite uneasy, because if Nick did not accept the lungs immediately, they would be offered to another recipient, and it would be extremely unlikely that he'd receive another chance. It took some gentle persuasion from his parents and even from me over the phone to convince him that this opportunity was well worth skipping a day at the beach, and he did finally agree to board a hastily arranged flight to the transplant center.

Nick's surgery was a success. A few months after he'd decided to give up, he was back in school full-time. He would go on to ride bikes, play with his friends, and take up new hobbies. He'd spend time with his parents, sisters, and big extended family and go on other vacations.

Transplanted lungs don't last forever, and the people who loved Nick most knew that one day his health would again deteriorate. But for the next several years, they embraced the gift of precious time with him and celebrated both the boy and the life he almost didn't have. As someone who endeavors to support families of sick children every day, I know no greater testament to any positive therapy than seeing a seed of hope help enable a child to go back to living as fully as possible at the heart of a loving family.

FAMILY DYNAMICS

Sometimes, in order for a child to heal, the process needs to start with addressing family dysfunction that's triggering their symptoms. This was the case for a boy and his mother who were struggling to create a healthy bedtime routine after years of anxiety and inadequate sleep. Aidan was twelve years old when I met him, and both he and his mom suffered from anxiety. When he was little, his mom had made a habit of lying down beside him so he'd feel comfortable falling asleep at bedtime. This nightly interaction also eased his mother's anxiety about leaving him alone in his bedroom. Years passed, though, and this routine became disruptive, because even if Aidan got up in the night to use the bathroom, he woke up his mother to help him get back to sleep because he didn't know how to do so on his own.

Both members of this little family wanted to create a new routine in which each slept in their own beds.

I explained to Aidan and his mother how his sleeping difficulties had been triggered and that the solution involved his mother leaving him at night and Aidan learning to fall asleep on his own. This required that both Aidan and his mother tolerate the discomfort of separation, which I assured them would get easier with time. I offered to teach Aidan how to use hypnosis to fall asleep more easily, but he said he thought he could handle the separation by himself. I accepted his brave assessment and instructed his mom that she should tuck him in at night, leave his room, and under no circumstances (except an emergency) return to his room or allow him to enter her room until morning. Both Aidan and his mother agreed to follow this plan.

Three days later, Aidan's mother emailed to let me know how distressed she'd become because Aidan cried each night and called for her. She was worried that his lack of sleep would affect his school performance. I reassured her that it would take him some time to readjust, but her most productive course of action was to stick with the plan.

Three weeks later at his follow-up, Aidan and his mother were still tired and unhappy from lack of sleep. This time, when I offered to teach Aidan how to help himself with hypnotic imagery, he was ready to learn. I taught him how he might imagine falling asleep in his relaxing place and suggested this would help him fall asleep in real life. The following evening and thereafter, Aidan no longer reported difficulties with falling or staying asleep. He and his mom were both free of their unhealthy codependent arrangement.

The solution to this problem required full participation not just from this child but also from his mom. Their work together to eliminate the triggers for his sleep issues succeeded because each agreed to help the other.

THE STUDENT BECOMES THE TEACHER

The impacts of hypnosis on patients and families can range from monumental moments like the ones I experienced with Nick and his family to small, reflective ones with patients who arrive with treatable problems, learn how to cure themselves, and move on with their lives. Even among these patients who may only spend a few hours in treatment, the reach of hypnosis to their families is clear.

One of my patients, Vanessa, was ten years old when she arrived with a bundle of anxiety-related behaviors likely brought on by a long history of bullying followed by the frustrations of coping with pandemic-related life changes. She was suffering from dizziness, nausea, stomachaches, shaking, and eczema that seemed to worsen when she'd been under stress. These were all likely functional symptoms, and I felt confident Vanessa could be cured of them by learning hypnosis to calm herself and live with more confidence.

Most remarkable about Vanessa's case was that she took a lesson learned during her first appointment and extended it to her family in the best possible way. Just days after that visit, her grandmother was diagnosed with breast cancer and underwent surgery to remove a tumor. Vanessa utilized the positive talk we'd practiced during her visit to help her entire family, especially her younger brother, cope with this situation. She told herself that her grandmother would be OK, that the tumor was small, and that it had been caught early. She processed that assessment from all the information she was hearing at home, and she made it her role to remind the family at every opportunity that there were many reasons to feel hopeful and positive about their future. At her next visit, I congratulated Vanessa for her excellent use of positive talk and taught her how to use hypnosis to calm herself. She found her relaxation place at a lake her family had visited on vacation, and she embraced the task of practicing going there in her mind and using her relaxation sign to ease her anxiety and the symptoms it was causing.

Vanessa's mother remarked that even a little bit of practice at hypnosis shifted her daughter's outlook from one in which she felt at the mercy of every aspect of her circumstances to one in which she believed she had her own sphere of influence.

"It couldn't have come at a better time," she said. "A month ago my mother's diagnosis would have sent Vanessa spinning into sickness and stress, but right now she's actually helping all of us."

Vanessa's experience is unique to her story, but many other children who learn to use hypnosis also choose to use their new empowerment to help others. I have had several patients who've shared stories of how they taught a friend or sibling to use positive talk during school or sports events. Others have shared how their own narratives of success inspired people in their orbit to make changes—like the patient who told me he helped his girlfriend increase her grades from Cs to As by guiding her to stay calm during tests. Children who have mastered their own self-regulation have become leaders among peers who are trying to quit drugs or find their way back from depressive episodes, and they're quicker to recognize when someone they care about needs professional help and to encourage them to seek it.

I frequently remind patients providing this kind of outreach to friends and family that they lack training. A number of them have in turn developed interest in becoming medical professionals, psychologists, and counselors. One young woman who sought help when she was seventeen and had missed a year of school because of debilitating headaches and abdominal pain became so firmly confident by using hypnosis to take charge of her own health that she went on to nursing school so she could help others.

WHAT YOU CAN DO ON YOUR OWN
One hallmark of progress in a child's mental or physical health is reaching a moment when they feel confident and strong enough to extend a helping hand to someone else. The act of helping another person helps a child recognize their own strength and influence. You can lean into this concept with the children in your life in a number of ways. In the simplest sense, when your child learns new skills—in hypnosis or another mind-body field or anything they feel good about—ask about

those skills and express appreciation of your child's emotional growth. Be open to learning new skills as a role model alongside your child and encourage your child to pursue any healthful activity that makes them feel capable and positive.

Another opportunity to engage your child's sense of capability arises anytime someone else in their family or circle of friends faces a challenge. Ask your child what they might be able to do to help and support them in following through. Taking on the role of looking out for another person is an empowering practice for kids of all ages.

Family dynamics can play a big role in children's lives. Disagreements or stress within the family can often affect the children, and this may cause development or worsening of physical and mental health symptoms. In such situations, consider seeking help from a family therapist who can help identify specific behaviors that might be changed, resolve conflicts, and improve communication within the family, including through learning how to listen better to one another.

V

HYPNOSIS PRINCIPLES IN ACTION

Putting It All Together

Seven Steps to Guide Children and Teens toward Strength and Wellness

Over the course of teaching hypnosis to thousands of children and observing the ways they've chosen to use it to better their lives, I've seen a few recurrent attitudes, shifts in perspective, and ways of approaching challenges emerge time and again. Each of these derives from the hypnosis process but is not necessarily uniquely tied to hypnosis. In other words, these are habits you can learn to develop through steps taken on your own. We can all, for example, use positive words or believe in our own power. Hypnosis helps us truly trust that these self-enhancements are possible, and it gently, consistently guides us back toward them.

Any child, whether or not they choose to use hypnosis, should feel good about embracing the steps in this chapter.

1. USE POSITIVE WORDS FOR POSITIVE THOUGHTS

Automobile manufacturer Henry Ford knew all about the power of positive talk. He said, "Whether you think you can or think you can't, you are right." This adage is true in how we think about ourselves, and it's also an important factor in how we think about and speak to others. Deliberately choosing positive words and corresponding positive thoughts is something anyone can do with great, even potentially life-changing results.

Usually, during the first session with new patients, I discuss the importance of positive self-talk as a prelude to the use of hypnosis. We explore how children telling themselves they are strong or weak actually translates into increased or decreased muscle strength. I physically demonstrate this concept when I ask them to resist me as I push down on their outstretched arms. We then consider that saying "I'm not weak" doesn't result in as much strength as saying "I'm strong"—because our mind focuses on the main word: *weak.*

A person choosing positive words does so with the understanding that the subconscious will focus on the main message we tell ourselves—and carry it out to the best of its abilities.

One of the reasons the power of positive talk works is that it helps the mind consider new possibilities. For example, a ten-year-old who had a falling out with some of her friends might react by saying to herself, *I'm never going to have friends. Nobody likes me.* When her mind hears these thoughts, it reacts with agreement—and this causes the girl to feel even worse. However, when this child says something that is absolutely true—and also positive—about the unfortunate situation, like *I want to make more friends and for them to like me,* her mind reacts with agreement but this time causes the girl to feel better.

How does it work? In the first scenario, with its negative words, all the power harnessed by the girl's subconscious—all the things she can do and say and believe—are directed to stand down, to give up. In the second scenario, the girl's mind is instead prompted to think, *How will I make new friends? How can I get people to like me? Maybe I should go to the playground to meet new kids. Maybe I should have a party and invite my classmates.* I remind my patients to remain positive as they evaluate new ideas that come to mind as a result of this process.

Positive talk can equally be a sort of antidote to other people's negativity. I explain to my patients that pessimistic comments expressed by others can incite a negative reaction in themselves. To counteract and protect themselves from such incoming negativity, I encourage them to practice using positive self-talk.

Encourage your child to regularly use positive self-talk, to say these things out loud, and to talk to themselves using their own name (in the third person). All of these tools can help the child feel empowered and confident. If they find this task awkward or difficult at first, there's a simple, effective way to reframe the exercise: Tell them to speak to themselves with the same tone, manner, and attitude they'd use to speak to a beloved friend.

2. BELIEVE IN YOUR POWER

One of the most important things I've learned while observing patients in hypnosis is that we each have a guiding power within us. Hypnosis opens a pathway to that power, but even without hypnosis, it is there. Encourage your child to sit quietly and trust their own wisdom, strength, and resilience. Albert Einstein recognized the importance of a tranquil mind when he said, "The monotony and solitude of a quiet life stimulates the creative mind."

In terms of practical application, this means choosing to trust yourself and believe in yourself. It means recognizing that you are capable of feeling better or performing better under your own direction and that you can bravely become involved in new activities. Every endeavor can be framed as a success—either accomplishing a goal or learning something valuable in the process of coming up short.

Sometimes we believe that who we are is what we do—how we spend our days, hours, and minutes. It's easy for anyone, especially a child, to believe habits and routines are just the way things are and that this defines their character, but the fact is that actions can be changed. For example, some children think that if they do something wrong, this means that they are inherently bad. I reframe this thinking by suggesting that each child is a good person who has made a mistake from which they can learn.

Another important way you can believe in your own power is in remembering that things that can be learned sometimes can be *un*learned. For example, research has shown that a patient can be tricked into developing an allergic reaction by being shown an artificial goldenrod plant. This reaction occurs because the patient has learned that goldenrod triggers her allergies, and her mind and body have learned to react even when there's no pollen present.[1] This is similar to Paul's reaction to the imagined cheeseburger that first set me on the path to learning about hypnosis.

As occurred with Paul, such psychological reactions can be unlearned.

I've had many patients overcome diagnoses as varied as vocal cord dysfunction, irritable bowel syndrome, fainting, and dyslexia once they realized they had the power within themselves to control their symptoms. This was likely because the persistence of these symptoms was related to anxiety, and hypnosis helps kids manage that trigger.

With or without hypnosis, believing you have power to control something that brings hardship into your life is the first step in overcoming or making peace with that difficulty.

3. BE INTENTIONAL

Intention is key to staying on the path toward a goal. Teach your child to focus their intention deliberately. Emphasize that doing well along a path is more important than achieving any particular goal. As long as the child can be productive and derive strength from their journey, goal achievement is of less importance. After all, once a goal is achieved, a new goal must be set in order to keep moving forward.

My best example of this may come from my own life. Years ago my doctor told me I needed to either lose weight or begin taking diabetes medications. I came to view the challenge to lose weight and wrest back control of my health as an opportunity to do the kind of work I encourage my patients to do every day—to demonstrate to myself and to them that I could use the skills I've learned from hypnosis to change my life.

The plan I came up with contained no secrets, just common sense and confidence that I could succeed. First, I chose to recognize that I had a problem. Second, I determined that I was capable of solving it. Up until that time, I'd been inclined to believe my weight issue and high cholesterol levels were hereditary problems—things I couldn't control. In fact, heredity was one small factor—certainly not the biggest one. The intention to define my health condition as just that—a condition rather than a part of who I was—meant I could modify it. With this in mind, I set my goal and determined the steps I would take to reach it (a process that took some homework and trial and error as I learned that moderate exercise and a small, consistent reduction in caloric intake were sufficient to reduce weight). I enlisted the support of my wife, doctor, and friends.

Lastly, I gave myself a suggestion—one my patients were proud to see me embrace. I decided to equate feeling *hungry* with two other "h" words: *happy* and *healthy*. There were times in the first weeks when I was feeling all three *h*s to the extreme, but I maintained the association, and it worked. At the end of six months, I'd corrected my weight and brought my body mass index into the ideal range.

In working toward physical and mental health goals, people rarely have perfect success. As with the difficulties most of us encounter when we choose to change the way we eat, we experience both progress and setbacks. What matters most is that we get up each morning, reset our positive intentions, and apply ourselves to seeing them through.

The important lesson I took from my own experience and have seen countless boys and girls learn in their own ways is that my intentions mattered—they shaped my success.

As kids face challenges, encourage them to set their intentions and be confident in them. If one approach to overcome a challenge isn't working, find another way. Create a more focused plan and embrace it. Intentions lead to confidence, positivity, and determination. Each of these elements will help pave the way to success and wellness.

4. SOOTHE YOURSELF

Parents and doctors often talk about teaching babies to self-soothe—the process by which children learn that they are independently capable of becoming comfortable and falling asleep. As children become older, as they go through their teens and enter adulthood, they need reminders that they still possess the skills to calm themselves and benefit from the power of a tranquil state.

The best time to work on self-soothing skills isn't in the middle of a crisis; it's a little bit every day, a few minutes of quiet "me time" during which kids practice reaching their personal, spiritual center. In hypnosis, this is often a specific and imagined geographic place—like Paul's lake. Even outside hypnosis, though, anyone can practice soothing techniques and, over time, train the body and mind to become more relaxed as a habit and at will. To accomplish this, use these steps to create your routine:

- Breathe deliberately. Engage the breath as a way of slowing down and becoming calm. In a quiet place, inhale slowly through your nose, counting to five while you do it. Now hold that breath for another count of five. Now exhale through your mouth, slowly, for another count of five. The number is just a guideline. The important thing is to think about your breathing and do it in a controlled manner. It is amazing how this simple step, repeated over a few moments, can physically and mentally recenter us and allow us to think clearly and calmly.
- Listening to soothing music while doing hypnosis can be very helpful. Listening to it as a self-calming ritual is also a valuable habit to establish. Over time, repeatedly using a soundtrack can create an association between the music and your mood—triggering a response just like an anchoring gesture. People do this all the time to rev up their energy, creating set lists that feature spirited songs to pace their workout or practice routines.
- Meditate. Meditation is a sister to hypnosis on the wellness continuum. While the two mind-body practices are not the same, they share the power to create calm and are amazing tools for self-soothing. How can a child meditate? One way is to learn by your example, but

kids often like to choose their own meditation resources, and there are many books, apps, and YouTube channels designed with this in mind. Encourage your child to try one and support their setting aside the time and energy to practice it regularly.

5. BE AN ACTIVE LISTENER AND ADVOCATE

When children and teens act in apparently irrational ways, there are nearly always underlying reasons, and once those reasons are addressed, things often improve. When family members learn to be active listeners, this can have an immediate impact on helping children express their thoughts, feelings, and insights about their own behavior.

Active listening goes beyond hearing what someone is saying into the territory of focusing, acknowledging, and empathizing. Active listening can be employed deliberately when the listener states their understanding of what the speaker just said. The speaker can either affirm this or restate their thought until the listener understands it. Active listening also can be facilitated when the listener asks clarifying questions of the speaker, thus demonstrating interest in what is being said.

Many times I've encountered families for whom this simple shift in communication changes relationships and eases or eliminates problems. For example, an eight-year-old boy was in the habit of locking the bathroom door in his busy household, sparking concerns and altercations with siblings and parents. When I asked this child why, he explained that he was afraid of monsters in the bathroom. This dialogue was the first time his mother heard that his behavior was based in fear. When I suggested the boy make "monster spray" to use in the bathroom, he agreed and said he didn't think he'd need to lock the door anymore. I gave him a recipe of commonly available household ingredients (water, salt, lemon juice, and cinnamon—because of course monsters *hate* cinnamon) to mix together and apply with a spray bottle at home, with one spray being effective for twenty-four hours.

That was the end of that particular problem for this family—it never came up again.

Interestingly, once parents become active listeners—as this child's mother did during and after the appointment—they also become more effective advocates for their children's needs. This small issue was dividing this family, but once they had a shared understanding and objective, they worked together to resolve it.

Active listening and advocacy go hand in hand. Once you better understand your child's needs, you will also better understand how to help and how to problem-solve with creative solutions. A family whose child required daily injections for a blood-clotting condition helped him learn to blow soap bubbles during the shot routine to cope and stay calm. Another child carried a comfort toy to regularly scheduled physical therapy appointments to feel like a friend was present. A student asked for and was granted permission to stand in the back of a classroom because doing so made it easier for her to self-manage her attention issues.

In each case, a parent not only helped the child arrive at a solution that worked but also educated a health care or teaching professional about the coping skill, why it was working, and why the child should be permitted to use it.

As a last benefit, being an actively listening parent sets an example for your children. They can learn how to become effective and empathetic communicators themselves—a life skill that will serve them well.

6. PRACTICE GRATITUDE

There is always something for which to be grateful. Instinct and science show us that living with gratitude graces us with better physical and mental health and stronger relationships.[2]

There are many ways to easily put this evidence into practice at home. Create a gratitude corkboard and get it started with a favorite family photo or a note about something you love, or put a gratitude jar on the counter and fill it with mementoes of things the family is grateful for. Start family meals (not just at Thanksgiving) by sharing something that makes you feel grateful.

In addition to encouraging children to show gratitude, express it yourself. Make it a habit to point out what you are grateful for and frequently, sincerely let your child know you are grateful for their presence in your life and why.

In my practice, I've often seen children who live with severe and chronic health issues learn to put their hardships in perspective by focusing on the things for which they are grateful.

7. BELIEVE IN SOMETHING BIG

Learning to believe in something bigger than themselves allows children to put life into better perspective and can help them find meaning. Kids can be taught to believe in something big by being exposed to natural wonders, great works of art and literature, or houses of worship. They can also be taught that their small voices from within can tap into the powers of the universe, which teaches them to look inward for strength and thus become more self-reliant.

Many teenagers are trying to figure out what they are going to do in life and worry if they don't have set goals and plans. I point out that the average person changes careers a number of times throughout life and tell them that I didn't find hypnosis—something critical to my life's work—until I was forty. Rather than feel they have to lay out their entire lives before them, kids can choose an early life goal and work toward it, while trusting that even if their goals change, they will continue to function within the bounds of a higher plan. The subconscious often tells kids when they are on the right track, but in order to find this inner reassurance, they must trust that they do have inner wisdom.

Some kids worry about whether God is real. This question provides an opportunity for parents to start a discussion about the fact that living life as if God is real can be helpful in terms of deciding what is right and wrong. This tentative belief allows children to effectively "try on" faith, and in my experience some find enough reassurance and comfort in it to continue down that path.

Regardless of where and how kids choose to believe in something bigger than themselves, those who do are able to see themselves as part of a large, powerful, and benevolent whole. They are able to recognize that as part of this entity, they themselves are exceptional and necessary. Kids who realize they are special are calmer about allowing life to unfold because they're able to trust that something good will occur.

23

Coping in Crisis

Seven Ways Parents Can Help Children Create Calm in a Storm

The steps in chapter 22 can all help children and adults feel stronger and more centered in their daily lives. There are inevitably times, though, when kids need something more. Children of all ages are capable of adjusting to hardships and making peace with traumas and embracing full, productive, and healthy lives. What it takes to reach that point, though, varies by child, family, and circumstance. Some kids seem to naturally gravitate toward a healthy center. Some have to learn how to get there. When you're living with a child in crisis, it can feel like nothing else matters. A child's pain, fear, and anxiety impact everyone in a family, and those families often feel there is little or no help available to them.

Many events can provoke a crisis in a child's life—for example, the divorce of their parents, the death of a loved one, a family's move to a new environment, a house fire, homelessness, severe bullying in school, dealing with a difficult adult, participating in or witnessing a violent incident, man-made or natural disasters, and war. Children can even develop significant problems as a result of exposure to traumatic events solely through media coverage.

Because it's an event that impacted children of all ages and backgrounds around the world, the 2020 pandemic shone a bright light on just how much conventional medicine has overlooked the psychological component of children's health. During a time when many of the things children and teens rely on to keep them steady during tumultuous and emotional periods shut down, the rates of hospital admissions for pediatric patients dealing with mental problems skyrocketed, up nearly 25 percent for children and more than 30 percent for teenagers.[1] These numbers do not include all the children who were treated for physical symptoms and released while they were still dealing with overwhelming psychological issues, or children who visited a family physician but not an emergency room, or the countless children who suffered significant distress but never sought help.

Not surprisingly, the children most vulnerable to struggling with anxiety, depression, anger, isolation, and functional health problems during the COVID crisis were the same kids who had already been mired in or on the precipice of these things before 2020. Certainly these children deserve far more thoughtful, thorough care than bandages and medications and the occasional twenty-four-hour psychiatric hold. They need care that teaches them how to cope with their feelings without reaching their crisis point.

In many circumstances there is no substitute for professional medical or psychological consultation to help your child, but, on an everyday basis, you can take steps to help foster kids' competence and confidence. There are ways you can empower them to learn to cope better with stress. The keys are in learning how to think in ways that let children calmly interpret stressful triggers. When a child can do that, triggers are much less likely to have intense physical or mental effects.

Each of the general wellness steps in chapter 22 is applicable to children facing tough times. I can think of no circumstance in which using positive talk, for example, or taking care of one's body isn't beneficial. In addition, the following steps can help kids learn to manage their feelings. In an ideal world, children can practice and strengthen these skills as they grow and mature. They are worthy of conversations long before a crisis. However, there is no time like the present to start gently sharing some of these concepts with children who are struggling or seem on the verge of losing their balance.

1. TAKE A STEP BACK

One of the great strengths of hypnosis is that it helps create distance between a crisis and a child's reactions to it. Stressful events can wreak havoc on our lives, causing pain and suffering, anxiety, depression, and physical illness. All of these symptoms can make it seem like there's no separating bad things that are happening in the environment from the person who is experiencing the difficult circumstances.

Parents can help children achieve degrees of separation from their problems by routinely reinforcing recognition that they do not need to internalize the effects of a stressful event. For example, children who were unharmed in a car accident can become traumatized by internalizing a realization that they could be injured in another accident. A healthier response would be to remain calm and focus on the fact that they are safe rather than the potential deleterious effects of the accident. The value of keeping stress at bay is vast because internalized stress can change how we're feeling and acting in ways that are basic to human biology. When a child is in the middle of a crisis and feeling overwhelmed, the body responds by increasing adrenaline and cortisol levels and allowing the fight-or-flight part of the brain to run the show. The results of this stress-driven state can include rash decision making, lashing out from anger or fear, and rejecting help.[2]

Getting even a little mental distance from a crisis, however, allows the brain to calm down, hormones to rebalance, and the reasoning centers in your child's brain to take the reins in their response. The result? More measured responses, more careful decision making, more logic and less raw emotion.

How can you help facilitate this distance? We often hear references to people spiraling down, or spiraling out of control, in difficult times. How much better would it be for us to help one another spiral up, back toward wellness and balance? Our children can learn to use their emotions on a path leading to healing, including recognizing that they may need help in dealing with some strong emotions. Here, again, the power of words comes into play, as they can be used to manage perspective and guide your child toward rational, healthy thought processes. For example:

- Use words that define the problem as a separate entity. Start by choosing words that identify the problem as something separate from the child. Helpful statements include "I wonder how different people react differently to the same event," "You can't control the event, but you can control your reactions to it," and "Your injury is physical, but you can decide how you want to react to it." Sometimes it helps to coach your child to distance from the problem by talking about it in the third person. A child named Chris might ask, "How does Chris think this problem might be solved?"
- Use words to shift the child's perspective to that of an outsider. Ask what your child might do to help a friend or beloved relative in the same circumstance they're suffering.
- Use words to paint a picture of an alternate way to deal with a crisis. For an angry child, this might be something as simple as saying, "Let's sit down at the table so you can tell me why you feel this way." For a child dealing with depression, it might start with an invitation to go for a walk or to the park—to go outside where the change in the light and the air can help shift a mood, at least temporarily. Each offer allows the child to visualize doing something different in the moment, which provides a little distance from raging emotions.
- Lastly, "take a deep breath" is a universal saying among parents and teachers for good reason. The simple act of deliberately, slowly inhaling and exhaling can change a child's focus from an external one to an internal one in seconds. Thinking about their own breathing draws children back to their own center and can help them find a reset when they need it most. Physiologically, these deep, controlled

breaths send an important message to the brain to calm the fight-or-flight response. Thus, taking ten measured, focused deep breaths can help deescalate many moments of crisis and help your child create an all-important feeling of perspective on a situation.

2. PRACTICE RELAXATION

Kids in crisis can learn to recenter themselves and achieve a sense of calm by practicing relaxation. In hypnosis, this is something kids learn to achieve at will, but at home you can support your child in finding other shortcuts to calm.

Focus on creating both a physical and a mental place to relax. The physical place can be a quiet outdoor spot, a favorite chair, a spot to curl up with a special pillow and blanket, or anywhere your child chooses. Encourage kids to combine using this physical location or position with mental images of a favorite relaxing moment, like the children in this book have done in hypnosis. Kids can "practice" feeling calm and centered in this space by reading a favorite book there or writing, sketching, or doing some other quiet activity they enjoy. Having quiet, positive moments in this place will help imbue it with a sense of wellness when the child needs help feeling calm.

Sometimes the greatest need for this kind of centering is when children are not at home or when they have limited opportunities to do it privately. In that case, your child can put together a comfort box or bag—a sort of to-go version of their relaxing space. I've known many children (and even some adults) who've been able to use this approach to help them achieve calm at school or at work. The logic is similar to that of having a worry stone or a lucky penny in your pocket—in this case, a talisman for calm.

One of my patients, a ten-year-old boy, made a comfort box he could open whenever he felt overwhelmed. He placed his favorite Pokemon card inside so he could look at it, two small Chinese Baoding stress balls that he could roll and jingle in his hand, and a small piece of a baby blanket he liked to hold. Next he added a small bag of favorite jelly beans that he could smell and taste. His box encompassed things that he loved, that made him feel comforted, and that engaged all of his senses. By interacting with its contents, he learned to calm himself with a tool of his own making.

3. REFRAME

It's a challenge for children and teens to find perspective, to be able to look at an event and put it in the context of a week, a month, a year, or an entire life. Most simply haven't had time to witness the fact that life has a rhythm of ups and downs and that even in our darkest times, there will be something to look forward to or be glad about again. It can also be difficult for kids to consider the context of the wider workings of the world. Their views tend to be narrow and self-involved—which is not a failing but a normal part of their development.

Parents, teachers, and clinicians can help children widen their view to thoughtfully put their troubles in context. As an example, consider my patient Cristobal, whom I'd known for several years before the COVID-19 pandemic. During that time, Cristobal made amazing strides in overcoming his anxiety and stuttering and in learning to accept the impacts and challenges brought to his life because of his cerebral palsy. Like so many people his age, in 2020 Cristobal was taking his first significant steps toward independence when the pandemic struck. He was going to college, living on campus, creating a new circle of friends, and tackling mature course work. Each of these accomplishments in Cristobal's life was hard earned. When his campus closed and he had to go home to a socially isolated life, he grieved what he perceived as the loss of the progress he'd made (not to mention the fun life he was creating on campus).

As the pandemic unfolded, Cristobal's sense of loss was compounded by his fears for himself, the people he cared about, the country, and the world at large. He worried about people getting sick and dying, about people losing their jobs, and about whether the government was responding appropriately and in everyone's best interest. All these emotions made the year he was home a test of Cristobal's creativity, resolve, and resilience.

Cristobal and I discussed his challenges at length, and eventually I asked if he could think of anything positive that might occur as a result of the pandemic. He was able to think of several, including that people would read more books as other sources of entertainment dried up, that board games might make a resurgence, and that families might have more opportunities to bond with each other. When we brainstormed a little more, he considered that more animals would be adopted from shelters into loving homes and that many people would grow to better appreciate the importance of good hygiene and the power of immunizations. We discussed how some people would discover new talents and skills and that many would find ways to work from home when that had not seemed possible before. We considered that this situation could especially be a boon to people with physical disabilities who have long struggled to find an equal playing field in the workplace, as the job market would be easier on them if they didn't have to commute or navigate the logistics of in-office situations. As an environmentally minded young man, Cristobal noted that air pollution levels were dropping, and as a result the ozone layer was beginning to re-form during quarantines—both good things for the Earth.

None of these outcomes made the pandemic go away or diminished or erased the pain it caused, but they did give Cristobal another, more appreciative way to think about a difficult time in his life. I have rarely seen a circumstance in which a child can't find some worthwhile meaning in a difficult situation, even something to be grateful for, if they think deeply about it.

In addition to reframing crises from a wider view in terms of their impact, you can help kids consider the possibility of seeing them in the context of history. It is very easy for children and teens, with their limited perspective on the world, to think that a stressful or traumatic moment in time is a be-all and end-all. They haven't had the opportunity to learn how time mitigates even some of our most difficult challenges and changes. Children can benefit from imagining how an incident will be remembered by their future selves in the larger context of their lives—in five years, or ten, or forty.

For patients who learn and utilize hypnosis, this particular angle of inquiry takes on unique significance. Many children, Cristobal among them, have been told by their subconscious that it is older than they are or even that it has existed in previous lives. These children are able to take comfort in the knowledge that a part of them has been through worse things in the past and that it survived and thrived.

Investigating positive outcomes of difficult and negative events is much more than a rose-colored-glasses exercise; it allows for a shift in perspective that opens us up to the possibility that the world is bigger than ourselves and that perhaps our view in a particular moment is limited. This shift can change a child's attitude from despair to hopefulness and anticipation of a better future.

4. REMEMBER WHO YOU ARE

It is always the person going through hardship who must determine the path through it. If you are guiding or supporting a child during difficult times, try to think of your role as helping that child find choices and perspective, not pushing them down a single path. One way to facilitate this delicate process is to encourage kids to feel confident in who they are and in their capabilities. After all, every child should feel comfortable in the role of the hero of their own story. A simple shift of perspective from *I am a victim of this* to *I am going to get through this* is an empowering one.

To facilitate this attitude shift, start by making a habit of sharing family stories of resilience and accomplishment. Talk about the grandmother or old aunt who rejected convention and accomplished something special or the great-grandfather who built his own house or saved a soldier on a battlefield. Tell them how their parents met or stories of their own brave, smart, or loving antics when they were younger. Each family story is a link to a shared past, and in times of trouble kids can turn to this narrative to help them feel better about who they are and what they are capable of achieving.

When your child is having a hard time, don't supply the narrative for how they got there. Ask them to tell the story by posing gentle, open-ended questions that let them share their thoughts. A simple "Why do you think you were so upset this morning?" or "What can we do about this problem?" is usually enough to get the ball rolling so you can begin to understand where the child is coming from.

Being the hero of one's own story decidedly does not mean living it alone. Remind your child that there is a full supporting cast standing by to offer love, support, and guidance. For kids, an important part of taking ownership of their troubles is asking for the help they need. You can remind your child that the simple act of saying, "I need help with . . ." is a positive step. Doing so acknowledges a problem, lets others know their needs, and tacitly opens the door to accepting help when it's offered. Remind your child that the people who care about them want to participate in their healing.

Many children who practice hypnosis are able to ask the subconscious to help, and they frequently receive useful advice from it. Even without a way to talk directly with the subconscious, children can be reassured that they have wise souls and that they can overcome hardships because they are strong and resilient.

5. ACCEPT YOUR WHOLE SELF

Children often face tremendous pressures to achieve, to perform, and to embody certain personality traits or even physical characteristics. These pressures can drive kids to crisis, especially when they don't align with the child's true self. This is all too common among teenagers, who face competing pressures from different people in their lives—parents, peers, teammates, boyfriends and girlfriends, and the world of academia. The resulting anxieties often compound existing problems for kids who are already struggling to figure out who they are and what they want in life. This is a moment when kids are particularly vulnerable to developing anxiety, experiencing depression, turning to drugs, and even entertaining suicidal thoughts.

Seemingly paradoxically, there is no value in trying to sweep away your child's anxieties, fears, and health concerns. In fact, it's a recipe for disaster because those problems continue to fester even when avoided, away from the light of conversation and, if necessary, treatment. Instead, this is a time when kids need support in learning to focus on their own priorities, when they need encouragement to feel good about themselves—even the parts of themselves that they find hard to love.

Too often I meet children who are afraid of or even despise something that is a part of them. Children who struggle with chronic health problems may feel they hate the part of them that isn't healthy. Children who struggle with drug abuse may fear their part that is prone to addiction. Children may feel guilt or shame about parts of their experience or even their thoughts as they grow and mature. Many are extremely harsh with themselves, feeling they're not smart, not motivated enough, not attractive, or not likeable. They fear that their peers will judge them to be unworthy of friendship. These children need to learn to believe in themselves and receive the support of their families and their true friends. I suggest that their true friends will not judge them, but rather be supportive and accept them as they are. I often remind kids of the Dr. Seuss quote "Those who mind don't matter and those who matter don't mind."

In some cases, learning how to embrace the whole self is a taller order than in others. My patient Katie was a thoughtful, intelligent seventeen-year-old, a beloved daughter and a devoted sister to her younger siblings. She also sported tattoos of a cross and a skull and crossbones on her left forearm. Tragically, she struggled with a narcotics addiction through most of her teenage years, and during that time she came to think of herself as having two different personalities. One of these was bright, funny, loving, and generous; the other was selfish, angry, destructive, and fatalistic. The Katie who first sought help despised the "dark" side of herself, and when she experienced setbacks and made mistakes, she'd blame it. Sometimes she'd start to feel she was powerless to fight back against such a strong, negative force. She said she wished she could make the bad part go away.

I reflected that the dark side was part of Katie and that, as part of her, it needed to be preserved, and I hoped she could make peace with it instead of trying to banish it. I told her about a *Star Trek* episode in which Captain Kirk is divided into two parts: the good and the evil. It turned out that Kirk's good part was gentle and kind but also meek and indecisive. His evil part was selfish and greedy but also strong and deliberate. The man who was a good captain was an amalgam of both. To be fully functional as a human being, I told Katie, she could integrate both parts of herself rather than rejecting either one.

Encouraging children to be more accepting of themselves starts at home, with the acceptance of their families. When a child expresses self-loathing, parents can help the child consider ways to improve and provide appreciation and encouragement to help their child modify their self-characterization. When a child errs, parents should avoid making generalizations such as "You always mess up" or "You're lazy." Such statements can be internalized by the child and become their reality. Instead, parents might state, "I believe you can fix this situation" or "I wonder how you can get your assignments done in time." Acceptance of your child includes brainstorming with them about how things might improve and welcoming their solutions.

6. DO SOMETHING, BIG OR SMALL
Benjamin Franklin wrote, "Trouble springs from idleness," an adage that most every parent has uttered in some form, some of us many times over. For children in crisis, taking actions they can control helps put them back in the driver's seat of their experience. There are many ways this can and should happen, but I advise parents to keep the following ones in mind—and encourage kids to embrace them.

- Follow a routine. A basic routine that includes sufficient sleep, healthy meals, some kind of exercise, and time outside is an achievable goal for children and one that creates a sense of normalcy in their days. When trouble arises, routine helps them know what do to when they don't know what to do. It encourages a one-foot-in-front-of-the-other mentality, which is a great start for any child dealing with physical or mental health issues. It's fine to break with routine from time to time, but when kids learn to be deliberate about it, they'll be able to have both routine and flexible time. As a parent, you can facilitate routine with family dinners at predictable times and household schedules that engage the kids as well as the adults.

- Choose something new. During the COVID-19 crisis, I spoke with many children about the hardships and opportunities created by living in the time of a pandemic. One piece of advice I offered many of them was to take some of the time they were not spending in regular school to learn something new. "Years from now when this is all behind us," I'd suggest, "wouldn't it be great if you could look back and say that you learned to cook or play an instrument or the basics of a new language or how to teach your dog to do tricks during COVID?" Many children took me up on this, challenging themselves to do something novel, and those who did took pride in their new projects, in their creativity, and in their accomplishments.

- Do something kind. It seems to be written in human DNA that doing something for others makes us feel good about ourselves. Katie struggled not only with her addiction but also with her isolation during the COVID quarantine. She felt invisible and unwanted, both common emotional fears among drug users. When she was able to get a job working in a shop in the very early mornings, I called her on several occasions when she was on her commute to work in order to remind her of her worth and help set her intentions for the day. Most days I asked her the same four questions: What was she grateful for? (Her answer always started with "my family.") What was she looking forward to? Had she been thinking about drugs? And what good deed did she have planned for the day? It was her good deeds that Katie most liked to talk about, both before and after she did them. I could hear the positive energy in her voice each time. There are a million ways to do a good deed—for a family member, a neighbor, someone at church, pets, wildlife, and perfect strangers. Encourage your child—and show them by example—to participate in this simple and life-affirming practice.

7. TRUST YOURSELF; TRUST YOUR FAMILY

It's difficult to go through life feeling alone, and children especially need to feel they've got the support of family and friends as they navigate their way from childhood to adulthood. Without trust, children can be surrounded by friends and family and yet seem lonely and lost. You can help your child develop trust—both in you and in themselves—by first learning to be trusting. As a parent, be a role model for development of a trusting relationship by doing your best to keep your word. Whenever possible, give your child repeated opportunities to show responsible behavior. When the child does something wrong, explore the reasons for their actions and invite your child's opinion regarding how they can do better. This is a tacit acknowledgment that the child is a separate, important person with their own feelings, opinions, and needs.

When you find opportunities, remind your children that they possess inner wisdom and that they can trust in their own abilities to calm themselves, make good choices, and achieve goals that are important to them.

When children falter and are struggling, they need extra support and the confidence that their family will stand by them and guide them. When a child is in crisis, this isn't always an easy thing to convey or to do. Sometimes you have to get creative or put in some extra time to make it work. Consider doing something outside the bounds of your regular routine with your child, like camping or taking a class together or participating in a community event. In my practice, I often offer patients food, soda, or tea to show them they are important to me outside the bounds of the formal doctor-patient relationship and to symbolically nourish them in addition to providing them with medical care. This gesture builds trust because it helps children understand that I care about them.

One of my favorite metaphors for the care a clinician, teacher, or parent can provide came about during a visit with a young teenager. Trevor had been struggling with anxiety and depression and chronic health problems for years but had found very little help available to him. Even as he was learning hypnosis, Trevor doubted himself and his ability to find a healthy new normal. We discussed this fear at length in his sessions, and I told him I was confident he was getting better, adding, "I'll believe in you until you're strong enough to believe in yourself."

He looked puzzled and then sad.

"I don't think it works that way," he said.

In the moment, a new metaphor presented itself, an idea and an image I hoped he could associate with the perception of steady improvement.

"When you break a bone," I asked, "how does a cast help?"

"It protects the bone," he answered, an unspoken *obviously* implied in his tone.

"Yes, but how exactly does the bone heal?"

Trevor thought about this a moment before responding. "The body heals it."

"So . . . what does the cast do?"

"It helps the bone stay in place."

"That's exactly right," I nodded. "For now, I will act as your cast. I'll stabilize you until your mind heals itself."

At this promise, Trevor gave me a wide and genuine smile, a rare gift from a child who'd been feeling adrift for such a long time.

"I like that," he said.

"I like it too. And I'm looking forward to it."

Those few moments gave Trevor an idea he could hold, one that trusted in his inner power, one that reassured him he was not alone, one that subtly implied his body and his doctor and the universe would all work in concert to help him get better. This was hypnosis in its simplest form—the planting of an idea that would grow and bloom and offer a child a way to first visualize and then realize a world in which he felt well.

If a child in your life is in crisis, this is something you can offer and on which you can follow through. Be the support. Your efforts can be multifaceted, encompassing supporting your child in recognizing a problem, in learning to view it as separate from who they are, in coming up with a plan to make life better, and in creating and following through on changes and new routines that make that possible. Your child will feel empowered to know that your strong, active presence is a steady, positive force—and that they don't have to go it alone.

Epilogue

As my first hypnosis patient and my partner in learning about the process and its potential, Paul embraced his therapy eagerly and energetically. He often talked about his plans for his life, its meaning, and how he wanted to help people. I suggested that perhaps his teaching me about hypnosis was part of his role in life, and he agreed. As we worked together, Paul and I realized we were both learning a lot about how the mind operates. We often discussed the idea that someday I would write about our work together in a book, and Paul said he was happy I was keeping detailed records of our experiences.

After several months of working together, Paul told me that hypnosis was often helpful to him when he needed to calm himself during asthma attacks. The most dramatic example of this process occurred when he inadvertently ate a milk-containing product. He was rushed to the emergency room with extreme breathing difficulties. His throat had swollen dramatically, and the physicians felt that Paul would again need to be placed on a ventilator in order to help him breathe. As they were preparing to insert the breathing tube into his throat, Paul told me that he became very upset. He felt as if his physicians didn't know what they were doing, and he was angry about having to once again be so uncomfortable while on a ventilator.

"I was desperate," he explained. "So I decided to go to my lake. I became very calm at the lake and my breathing eased. Suddenly, I realized that there was no tube in my throat. I came out of hypnosis, and the doctors told me I was better. They said they didn't understand how I'd improved, but just as they were ready to put the tube in, my throat opened up.

"They had no idea what happened. But I knew," he concluded with a wink.

On one occasion, Paul's subconscious offered to handwrite a poem:

> *In the event of my demise*
> *When my heart can beat no more*
> *I hope I die for a principle*
> *Or belief I have lived for.*
>
> *I will die before my time*
> *Because I feel the shadow's depth*
> *So much I wanted to accomplish*
> *Before I reached my death.*
>
> *I have come to grips with the possibility*
> *And wiped the last tears from my eyes*
> *I loved all who were positive*
> *In the event of my demise.*

When he came out of hypnosis, Paul disavowed knowledge of this poem. He didn't understand how it came to be written. I wondered whether this is how people suddenly develop moments of inspiration. Perhaps a problem is worked out in their subconscious, and then the answer is delivered whole into awareness.

"Do you know what the poem means?" I asked.

"I think it shows a fear of dying young or unexpectedly," he replied. "Could we find out what my subconscious thinks?"

"Sure," I said. "Why don't you let your subconscious tell us?"

Moments later, Paul's subconscious wrote, *About dying unexpectedly and fading out like a dim bulb.*

"What does the poem mean by saying 'I hope I die for a principle or belief I have lived for'?" Paul asked.

I found it a little disconcerting to serve as an intermediary between him and his subconscious. Nevertheless I said, "OK, can you tell us what you meant by that line?"

Such as Malcolm X, Martin Luther King, they taught "you can kill a revolutionary but you cannot kill a revolution." He wants to make a statement about something.

"What does 'shadow's depth' mean?" I asked.

Been in the situation before, and shadows over me every time I get sick or go to the doctor and every time I get sick the shadow gets bigger and darker, that is why the bulb is fading.

I asked, "Should Paul be scared by this?"

Yes, because the shadow is big and dark.

I wondered whether Paul's concern about the "shadow's depth" was inhibiting him in some way. I thought that perhaps with use of hypnosis we could "lift" the shadows and make him feel better. So I asked his subconscious, "Does awareness of the shadow's depth inhibit Paul?"

No—contrary, it pushes him and makes him drive to improve himself in every aspect, specifically health-wise.

I understood this statement to mean that the shadow's depth was helpful to Paul. Perhaps this was one reason that he became my eager partner in exploration of hypnosis.

When Paul's health failed, I lost not only a patient but also a dear friend. The day before his funeral, I met with his parents at their home to thank them for allowing me to work with him. I told them their son had helped launch a new phase of my medical career. I said, "I want you to know I feel that when I help patients with hypnosis, this is an extension of Paul's work on this earth. In this way, I will help Paul live on. His work will be my work."

That day, I brought along the only audio tape we'd made during our work together, which was recorded on the day I first spoke with Paul's subconscious. I told Paul's parents I thought he would have wanted them to hear it, because he'd hope it would give them comfort.

On the recording, as his subconscious talks from the safety of his lake, Paul shares prophetic and healing observations about his life with his grieving family.

When I ask him on the tape who is with him in his relaxing place, Paul's subconscious answers, "Everyone important in my life, dead or alive, is with me."

Paul's subconscious describes visiting heaven in a dream. "Everyone is friendly, and everyone knows everyone. They're helpful and carefree. You don't have to worry about problems, suffering, or any earthly cares or worries. Everything happens naturally there. It's naturally good. I saw many of my relatives. There was a light. They were all sitting on a porch of a big white mansion. My grandmother said to me, 'It'll be all right.' My aunt said to me, 'You've beat the odds before, kid. You can do it again.' And God said, 'It will be okay, you are in My hands.'"

I often reflect that one of the many thanks I owe Paul is for entering into the exploration of hypnosis with me with the purest intentions—to learn, to teach, to heal, and to understand. Because of the push he gave me and the positive start we created together, thousands of patients who might otherwise have continued to suffer have found healing.

A Final Note about Hypnosis

I learned about vocal cord dysfunction (VCD) in 1998, just after I learned about hypnosis. This discovery occurred fifteen years after VCD was first described in a 1983 article that appeared in the *New England Journal of Medicine*.[1]

Even though I trained as a pediatric pulmonologist and had practiced in the field for nearly a decade, I had never realized that this diagnosis existed—and therefore had no idea about how I might treat patients with the condition. I'm positive that I saw patients with VCD before I learned about the diagnosis, but I likely attributed their shortness of breath to asthma, allergies, or gastroesophageal reflux. At that point in my career, I hadn't even considered anxiety as a likely cause of respiratory symptoms.

The VCD story illustrates a problem in the medical field: the incredibly slow dissemination of new information. This is especially true when there is no drug involved—and thus no pharmaceutical company publicizing a new medical condition or treatment option.

I think the slow uptake of hypnosis as an important therapy suffers similarly from the plodding pace at which physicians recognize and then embrace new information or paradigms that can lead to improved health outcomes. For example, even though hypnosis was recognized by major medical organizations in the 1950s as an effective tool in the management of pain, this fact was never taught to me when I attended medical school thirty years later. Even when I started my work with hypnosis in the late 1990s, one of my colleagues told me that I should not tell people that I used hypnosis, because I'd be labeled a "voodoo doctor."

I like to think that if a parent had come to me early in my pulmonary career and asked me whether I thought their child could be suffering from VCD, I'd have researched the diagnosis and thus accelerated my ability to diagnose and treat the condition. Even then, I believed that following my patients' leads was one of the most useful techniques at my disposal.

As we cannot depend on the medical system to efficiently spread the word about hypnosis, my hope is that parents who read this book will introduce the concept of hypnosis to their medical providers and thus start a grassroots movement that will accelerate its uptake as an invaluable resource for our children and society for generations to come.

Notes

CHAPTER 2

1. Hovec, Frank J. Mac. 1975. "Hypnosis Before Mesmer." *American Journal of Clinical Hypnosis* 17 (4): 215–220. https://doi.org/10.1080/00029157.1975.1 0403747.

2. Flynn, Niamh. 2018. "Systematic Review of the Effectiveness of Hypnosis for the Management of Headache." *International Journal of Clinical and Experimental Hypnosis* 66 (4): 343–352. https://doi.org/10.1080/00207144.20 18.1494432; Palsson, Olafur S. 2015. "Hypnosis Treatment of Gastrointestinal Disorders: A Comprehensive Review of the Empirical Evidence." *American Journal of Clinical Hypnosis* 58 (2): 134–158. https://doi.org/10.1080/00029 157.2015.1039114; Jacknow, Dale S., Jeanne M. Tschann, Michael P. Link, and W. Thomas Boyce. 1994. "Hypnosis in the Prevention of Chemotherapy-Related Nausea and Vomiting in Children: A Prospective Study." *Journal of Developmental and Behavioral Pediatrics* 15 (4): 258–264. https://doi.org/ 10.1097/00004703-199408000-00007; Keuthen, Nancy J., Richard L. O'Sullivan, Paige Goodchild, Dayami Rodriguez, Michael A. Jenike, and Lee Baer. 1998. "Retrospective Review of Treatment Outcome for 63 Patients with Trichotillomania." *American Journal of Psychiatry* 155 (4): 560–561. https://doi.org/10.1176/ajp.155.4.560; Vlieger, Arine M., Carla Menko-Frankenhuis, Simone C. S. Wolfkamp, Ellen Tromp, and Marc A. Benninga. 2007. "Hypnotherapy for Children with Functional Abdominal Pain or

Irritable Bowel Syndrome: A Randomized Controlled Trial." *Gastroenterology* 133 (5): 1430–1436. https://doi.org/10.1053/j.gastro.2007.08.072; Lazarus, Jeffrey, and Susan K. Klein. 2006. "Treatment of Tics in Patients with Tourette Syndrome with Self-Hypnosis Training Enhanced with Videotapes." *Journal of Developmental & Behavioral Pediatrics* 27 (5): 444–445. https://doi.org/10.1097/00004703-200610000-00063.

3. Jiang, Heidi, Matthew P. White, Michael D. Greicius, Lynn C. Waelde, and David Spiegel. 2017. "Brain Activity and Functional Connectivity Associated with Hypnosis." *Cerebral Cortex* 27 (8): 4083–4093. https://doi.org/10.1093/cercor/bhw220; Raz, Amir, Theodore Shapiro, Jin Fan, and Michael I. Posner. 2002. "Hypnotic Suggestion and the Modulation of Stroop Interference." *Archives of General Psychiatry* 59 (12): 1155. https://doi.org/10.1001/archpsyc.59.12.1155; Cojan, Yann, Lakshmi Waber, Sophie Schwartz, Laurent Rossier, Alain Forster, and Patrik Vuilleumier. 2009. "The Brain Under Self-Control: Modulation of Inhibitory and Monitoring Cortical Networks During Hypnotic Paralysis." *Neuron* 62 (6): 862–875. https://doi.org/10.1016/j.neuron.2009.05.021.

4. Barber, Theodore Xenophon, and David Smith Calverley. 1963. "'Hypnotic-Like' Suggestibility in Children and Adults." *Journal of Abnormal and Social Psychology* 66 (6): 589–597. https://doi.org/10.1037/h0041709; Poulsen, Bruce C., and William J. Matthews. 2003. "Correlates of Imaginative and Hypnotic Suggestibility in Children." *Contemporary Hypnosis* 20 (4): 198–208. https://doi.org/10.1002/ch.278.

5. Kravis, Nathan M. 1988. "James Braid's Psychophysiology: A Turning Point in the History of Dynamic Psychiatry." *American Journal of Psychiatry* 145 (10): 1191–1206.

CHAPTER 3
1. Yang, Seoyon, and Min Cheol Chang. 2019. "Chronic Pain: Structural and Functional Changes in Brain Structures and Associated Negative Affective States." *International Journal of Molecular Sciences* 20 (13). https://doi.org/10.3390/ijms20133130.

CHAPTER 4

1. Anbar, Ran D., and D. A. Hehir. 2000. "Hypnosis as a Diagnostic Modality for Vocal Cord Dysfunction." *Pediatrics* 106 (6): e81–81. https://doi.org/10.1542/peds.106.6.e81; Anbar, Ran D. 2001. "Self-Hypnosis for Management of Chronic Dyspnea in Pediatric Patients." *Pediatrics* 107 (2): e21–21. https://doi.org/10.1542/peds.107.2.e21.

2. Fretzayas, Andrew, Maria Moustaki, Ioanna Loukou, and Konstantinos Douros. 2017. "Differentiating Vocal Cord Dysfunction from Asthma." *Journal of Asthma and Allergy* 10 (October): 277–283. https://doi.org/10.2147/jaa.s146007.

CHAPTER 5

1. Proverbs 16:24.

2. Proverbs 18:21.

3. Lodge, Jackie, Diana Kim Harte, and Gail Tripp. 1998. "Children's Self-Talk Under Conditions of Mild Anxiety." *Journal of Anxiety Disorders* 12 (2): 153–176. https://doi.org/10.1016/s0887-6185(98)00006-1.

4. Newberg, Andrew B, and Mark Robert Waldman. 2013. *Words Can Change Your Brain: 12 Conversation Strategies to Build Trust, Resolve Conflict, and Increase Intimacy.* New York: A Plume Book.

5. Levine, Jon D., Newton C. Gordon, Richard Smith, and Howard L. Fields. 1981. "Analgesic Responses to Morphine and Placebo in Individuals with Postoperative Pain." *Pain* 10 (3): 379–389. https://doi.org/10.1016/0304-3959(81)90099-3; Kaptchuk, Ted J., Elizabeth Friedlander, John M. Kelley, M. Norma Sanchez, Efi Kokkotou, Joyce P. Singer, Magda Kowalczykowski, Franklin G. Miller, Irving Kirsch, and Anthony J. Lembo. 2010. "Placebos Without Deception: A Randomized Controlled Trial in Irritable Bowel Syndrome." Edited by Isabelle Boutron. *PLoS ONE* 5 (12): e15591. https://doi.org/10.1371/journal.pone.0015591; Benedetti, Fabrizio, Giuliano Maggi, Leonardo Lopiano, Michele Lanotte, Innocenzo Rainero, Sergio Vighetti, and Antonella Pollo. 2003. "Open Versus Hidden Medical Treatments:

The Patient's Knowledge About a Therapy Affects the Therapy Outcome."
Prevention & Treatment 6 (1), Article 1a. https://doi.org/10.1037/1522-3736.6.1.61a.

CHAPTER 7

1. Olness, Karen, John Macdonald, and D. L. Uden. 1987. "Comparison of Self-Hypnosis and Propranolol in the Treatment of Juvenile Classic Migraine." *Pediatrics* 79 (4): 593–597; Kohen, Daniel P., and Karen Olness. 2011. *Hypnosis and Hypnotherapy with Children*. New York: Routledge; Elkins, Gary, William Fisher, Aimee Johnson, and Jim Sliwinski. 2012. "Clinical Hypnosis for the Palliative Care of Cancer Patients." *Oncology* 26 (8): 26–30; Patterson, David R., John J. Everett, G. Leonard Burns, and Janet A. Marvin. 1992. "Hypnosis for the Treatment of Burn Pain." *Journal of Consulting and Clinical Psychology* 60 (5): 713–717. https://doi.org/10.1037/0022-006x.60.5.713.

CHAPTER 8

1. Bodde, N. M. G., J. L. Brooks, G. A. Baker, P. A. J. M. Boon, J. G. M. Hendriksen, and A. P. Aldenkamp. 2009. "Psychogenic Non-epileptic Seizures—Diagnostic Issues: A Critical Review." *Clinical Neurology and Neurosurgery* 111 (1): 1–9. https://doi.org/10.1016/j.clineuro.2008.09.028.

2. Dikel, William, and Karen Olness. 1980. "Self-Hypnosis, Biofeedback, and Voluntary Peripheral Temperature Control in Children." *Pediatrics* 66 (3): 335–340; Martínez-Taboas, Alfonso. 2002. "The Role of Hypnosis in the Detection of Psychogenic Seizures." *American Journal of Clinical Hypnosis* 45 (1): 11–20. https://doi.org/10.1080/00029157.2002.10403493.

3. Olson, Donald M., Neva Howard, and Richard J. Shaw. 2008. "Hypnosis-Provoked Nonepileptic Events in Children." *Epilepsy & Behavior* 12 (3): 456–459. https://doi.org/10.1016/j.yebeh.2007.12.003.

4. Anbar, Ran D. 2014. "Hypnosis for Children with Chronic Disease." In William C. Wester and Laurence I. Sugarman (eds.), *Therapeutic Hypnosis with Children and Adolescents*. 2nd ed. Carmarthen, UK: Crown House Publishing, 403–431.

5. Thomson, Linda. 2011. *Harry the Hypno-potamus: Metaphorical Tales for the Treatment of Children.* Carmarthen, UK: Crown House Publishing.

CHAPTER 9
1. Wagner, K. D. 2009. "Anxiety Disorders in Children and Adolescents: New Findings." *Psychiatric Times* 32 (3): 483–524.

CHAPTER 10
1. Jardine, David L., Wouter Wieling, Michele Brignole, Jacques W. M. Lenders, Richard Sutton, and Julian Stewart. 2018. "The Pathophysiology of the Vasovagal Response." *Heart Rhythm* 15 (6): 921–929. https://doi.org/10.1016/j.hrthm.2017.12.013.

CHAPTER 11
1. Bargh, John A., and Ezequiel Morsella. 2008. "The Unconscious Mind." *Perspectives on Psychological Science* 3 (1): 73–79. https://doi.org/10.1111/j.1745-6916.2008.00064.

2. Shenefelt, Philip D. 2011. "Ideomotor Signaling: From Divining Spiritual Messages to Discerning Subconscious Answers During Hypnosis and Hypnoanalysis, a Historical Perspective." *American Journal of Clinical Hypnosis* 53 (3): 157–167. https://doi.org/10.1080/00029157.2011.10401754.

3. Anbar, Ran D. 2001. "Automatic Word Processing: A New Forum for Hypnotic Expression." *American Journal of Clinical Hypnosis* 44 (1): 27–36. https://doi.org/10.1080/00029157.2001.10403453.

4. Anbar, Ran D., and Julie H. Linden. 2010. "Understanding Dissociation and Insight in the Treatment of Shortness of Breath with Hypnosis: A Case Study." *American Journal of Clinical Hypnosis* 52 (4): 263–273. https://doi.org/10.1080/00029157.2010.10401731.

CHAPTER 12
1. Anbar, Ran D., and Howard R. Hall. 2004. "Childhood Habit Cough Treated with Self-Hypnosis." *Journal of Pediatrics* 144 (2): 213–217. https://doi.org/10.1016/j.jpeds.2003.10.041.

CHAPTER 13

1. Anbar, Ran D. 2014. "Hypnosis for Children with Chronic Disease." In William C. Wester and Laurence I. Sugarman (eds.), *Therapeutic Hypnosis with Children and Adolescents* (403–431). 2nd ed. Carmarthen, UK: Crown House Publishing.

2. "Free Hypnosis to Be More Creative." Melbourne Hypnotherapy Clinic. https://melbournehypnotherapyclinic.com/free-hypnosis-be-more-creative; "Hypnotherapy for Highly Creative People." Browning Clinical Hypnotherapy. https://browninghypnotherapy.com/hypnotherapy-for-highly-creative-people-3; Creative Hypnosis: https://creativehypnosis.net.

3. Stuckey, Heather L., and Jeremy Nobel. 2010. "The Connection Between Art, Healing, and Public Health: A Review of Current Literature." *American Journal of Public Health* 100 (2): 254–263. https://doi.org/10.2105/ajph.2008.156497; Stickley, Theodore, Nicola Wright, and Mike Slade. 2018. "The Art of Recovery: Outcomes from Participatory Arts Activities for People Using Mental Health Services." *Journal of Mental Health* 27 (4): 367–373. https://doi.org/10.1080/09638237.2018.1437609.

4. Zhu, Junjia, Muhammad Hussain, Aditya Joshi, Cristina I. Truica, Darya Nesterova, Jolene Collins, Erika F. H. Saunders, Michael Hayes, Joseph J. Drabick, and Monika Joshi. 2020. "Effect of Creative Writing on Mood in Patients with Cancer." *BMJ Supportive & Palliative Care* 10 (1): 64–67. doi:10.1136/bmjspcare-2018-001710Zhu; Trauger-Querry, Barbara, and Katherine Ryan Haghighi. 1999. "Balancing the Focus: Art and Music Therapy for Pain Control and Symptom Management in Hospice Care." *Hospice Journal* 14 (1): 25–38. https://doi.org/10.1080/0742-969x.1999.11882912; Heenan, Deirdre. 2006. "Art as Therapy: An Effective Way of Promoting Positive Mental Health?" *Disability & Society* 21 (2): 179–191. https://doi.org/10.1080/09687590500498143.

5. Bailey, Lucanne Magill. 1986. "Music Therapy in Pain Management." *Journal of Pain and Symptom Management* 1 (1): 25–28. https://doi.org/10.1016/s0885-3924(86)80024-0; Smyth, Joshua M. 1998. "Written Emotional Expression: Effect Sizes, Outcome Types, and Moderating Variables." *Journal of Consulting and Clinical Psychology* 66 (1): 174–184. https://doi.org/10.1037/0022-006x.66.1.174.

6. Smith, Helen E., Christina J. Jones, Matthew Hankins, Andy Field, Alice Theadom, Richard Bowskill, Rob Horne, and Anthony J. Frew. 2015. "The Effects of Expressive Writing on Lung Function, Quality of Life, Medication Use, and Symptoms in Adults with Asthma." *Psychosomatic Medicine* 77 (4): 429–437. https://doi.org/10.1097/psy.0000000000000166.

CHAPTER 14

1. Linden, Julie H., Anuj Bhardwaj, and Ran D. Anbar. 2006. "Hypnotically Enhanced Dreaming to Achieve Symptom Reduction: A Case Study of 11 Children and Adolescents." *American Journal of Clinical Hypnosis* 48 (4): 279–289. https://doi.org/10.1080/00029157.2006.10401535.

2. Anbar, Ran D. 2001. "The Closure and the Rings: When a Physician Disregards a Patient's Wish." *Pediatric Pulmonology* 31 (1): 76–79.

3. Linden et al., "Hypnotically Enhanced Dreaming," 279–289.

CHAPTER 15

1. "Stuck in Denial? How to Move On." Mayo Clinic. 2017. https://www.mayoclinic.org/healthy-lifestyle/adult-health/in-depth/denial/art-20047926; Sher, Heather. 2019. "The Grace of Denial." *New England Journal of Medicine* 380 (2): 118–119. https://doi.org/10.1056/nejmp1810685.

2. White, Mathew P., Ian Alcock, James Grellier, Benedict W. Wheeler, Terry Hartig, Sara L. Warber, Angie Bone, Michael H. Depledge, and Lora E. Fleming. 2019. "Spending at Least 120 Minutes a Week in Nature Is Associated with Good Health and Wellbeing." *Scientific Reports* 9 (1). https://doi.org/10.1038/s41598-019-44097-3; "Sour Mood Getting You Down? Get Back to Nature." Harvard Health Publishing. July 2018. https://www.health.harvard.edu/mind-and-mood/sour-mood-getting-you-down-get-back-to-nature.

CHAPTER 16

1. Anbar, Ran D. 2008. "Subconscious Guided Therapy with Hypnosis." *American Journal of Clinical Hypnosis* 50 (4): 323–334. https://doi.org/10.1080/00029157.2008.10404299.

2. Anbar, Ran D., and Julie H. Linden. 2010. "Understanding Dissociation and Insight in the Treatment of Shortness of Breath with Hypnosis: A Case Study." *American Journal of Clinical Hypnosis* 52 (4): 263–273. https://doi.org/10.1080/00029157.2010.10401731; MacPhee, Edward. 2013. "Dissociative Disorders in Medical Settings." *Current Psychiatry Reports* 15 (10). https://doi.org/10.1007/s11920-013-0398-8.

3. Anbar, Ran D. 2004. "Stressors Associated with Dyspnea in Childhood: Patients' Insights and a Case Report." *American Journal of Clinical Hypnosis* 47 (2): 93–101. https://doi.org/10.1080/00029157.2004.10403628.

4. Anbar and Linden, "Subconscious Guided Therapy," 323–334.

CHAPTER 17

1. Vermeire, E., H. Hearnshaw, P. Royen, and J. Denekens. "Patient Adherence to Treatment: Three Decades of Research: A Comprehensive Review." *Journal of Clinical Pharmacy and Therapeutics* 26 (2001): 331–342.

2. Anbar, Ran D. 2001. "Self-Hypnosis for Management of Chronic Dyspnea in Pediatric Patients." *Pediatrics* 107 (2): e21–21. https://doi.org/10.1542/peds.107.2.e21.

3. Anbar, Ran D. 2000. "Of Mind, Body, and Modern Technology." *Clinical Pediatrics* 39 (7): 433–436. https://doi.org/10.1177/000992280003900711.

CHAPTER 18

1. Otgaar, Henry, Mark L. Howe, Lawrence Patihis, Harald Merckelbach, Steven Jay Lynn, Scott O. Lilienfeld, and Elizabeth F. Loftus. 2019. "The Return of the Repressed: The Persistent and Problematic Claims of Long-Forgotten Trauma." *Perspectives on Psychological Science* 14 (6): 1072–1095. https://doi.org/10.1177/1745691619862306.

2. Brunet, Alain, Daniel Saumier, Aihua Liu, David L. Streiner, Jacques Tremblay, and Roger K. Pitman. 2018. "Reduction of PTSD Symptoms with Pre-reactivation Propranolol Therapy: A Randomized Controlled Trial." *American Journal of Psychiatry* 175 (5): 427–433. https://doi.org/10.1176/appi.ajp.2017.17050481.

3. White, Rachel E., and Stephanie M. Carlson. 2015. "What Would Batman Do? Self-Distancing Improves Executive Function in Young Children." *Developmental Science* 19 (3): 419–426. https://doi.org/10.1111/desc.12314.

CHAPTER 19

1. Kentor, Rachel A., and Julie B. Kaplow. 2020. "Supporting Children and Adolescents Following Parental Bereavement: Guidance for Health-Care Professionals." *The Lancet Child & Adolescent Health* 4 (12): 889–898. https://doi.org/10.1016/s2352-4642(20)30184-x.

2. Hammond, D. Corydon. 2007. "Review of the Efficacy of Clinical Hypnosis with Headaches and Migraines." *International Journal of Clinical and Experimental Hypnosis* 55 (2): 207–219. https://doi.org/10.1080/00207140601177921.

CHAPTER 20

1. Anbar, Ran D. 2008. "Treatment of Psychological Complications of Prematurity with Self-Hypnosis: A Case Report." *Clinical Pediatrics* 48 (1): 106–108. https://doi.org/10.1177/0009922808322303.

2. Tillmann, Suzanne, Danielle Tobin, William Avison, and Jason Gilliland. 2018. "Mental Health Benefits of Interactions with Nature in Children and Teenagers: A Systematic Review." *Journal of Epidemiology and Community Health* 72 (10): 958–966. https://doi.org/10.1136/jech-2018-210436.

3. Lippi, Donatella. 2010. "Music and Medicine." *Journal of Multidisciplinary Healthcare* 137 (August). https://doi.org/10.2147/jmdh.s11378; Kemper, Kathi J., and Suzanne C. Danhauer. 2005. "Music as Therapy." *Southern Medical Journal* 98 (3): 282–288. https://doi.org/10.1097/01.smj.0000154773.11986.39.

4. Aknin, Lara B., Julia W. Van de Vondervoort, and J. Kiley Hamlin. 2018. "Positive Feelings Reward and Promote Prosocial Behavior." *Current Opinion in Psychology* 20 (April): 55–59. https://doi.org/10.1016/j.copsyc.2017.08.017.

CHAPTER 21

1. Pickles, Diane M., Stacey L. Lihn, Thomas F. Boat, and Carole Lannon. 2020. "A Roadmap to Emotional Health for Children and Families with

Chronic Pediatric Conditions." *Pediatrics* 145 (2) (February): E20191324. https://doi.org/10.1542/peds.2019-1324.

2. Anbar, Ran D. 2000. "Hypnosis, Theodore Roosevelt, and the Patient with Cystic Fibrosis." *Pediatrics* 106 (2): 339–339. https://doi.org/10.1542/peds.106.2.339.

3. Anbar, Ran D., and Vaani V. Murthy. 2010. "Reestablishment of Hope as an Intervention for a Patient with Cystic Fibrosis Awaiting Lung Transplantation." *Journal of Alternative and Complementary Medicine* 16 (9): 1007–1010. https://doi.org/10.1089/acm.2010.0107.

CHAPTER 22

1. Metzger, Frank C. 1947. "Emotions in the Allergic Individual." *American Journal of Psychiatry* 103 (5): 697–699. https://doi.org/10.1176/ajp.103.5.697.

2. Allen, Summer. 2018. *The Science of Gratitude* (Berkeley: Greater Good Science Center at University of California, Berkeley). https://ggsc.berkeley.edu/images/uploads/GGSC-JTF_White_Paper-Gratitude-FINAL.pdf.

CHAPTER 23

1. Leeb, R. T., R. H. Bitsko, L. Radhakrishnan, P. Martinez, R. Njai, and K. M. Holland. 2020. "Mental Health–Related Emergency Department Visits Among Children Aged <18 Years During the COVID-19 Pandemic—United States, January 1–October 17, 2020." *CDC Morbidity and Mortality Weekly Report* 69: 1675–1680.

2. Gilgoff, Rachel, Leena Singh, Kadiatou Koita, Breanna Gentile, and Sara Silverio Marques. 2020. "Adverse Childhood Experiences, Outcomes, and Interventions." *Pediatric Clinics of North America* 67 (2): 259–273. https://doi.org/10.1016/j.pcl.2019.12.001.

A FINAL NOTE ABOUT HYPNOSIS

1. Christopher, Kent L., Raymond P. Wood, R. Christa Eckert, Florence B. Blager, Roy A. Raney, and Joseph F. Souhrada. 1983. "Vocal-Cord Dysfunction Presenting as Asthma." *New England Journal of Medicine* 308 (26): 1566–70. https://doi.org/10.1056/nejm198306303082605.

Bibliography

Aknin, Lara B., Julia W. Van de Vondervoort, and J. Kiley Hamlin. 2018. "Positive Feelings Reward and Promote Prosocial Behavior." *Current Opinion in Psychology* 20 (April): 55–59. https://doi.org/10.1016/j.copsyc.2017.08.017.

Allen, Summer. 2018. *The Science of Gratitude.* Berkeley: Greater Good Science Center at University of California, Berkeley. https://ggsc.berkeley.edu/images/uploads/GGSC-JTF_White_Paper-Gratitude-FINAL.pdf.

Anbar, Ran D. 2000. "Hypnosis, Theodore Roosevelt, and the Patient with Cystic Fibrosis." *Pediatrics* 106 (2): 339–339. https://doi.org/10.1542/peds.106.2.339.

Anbar, Ran D. 2000. "Of Mind, Body, and Modern Technology." *Clinical Pediatrics* 39 (7): 433–436. https://doi.org/10.1177/000992280003900711.

Anbar, Ran D. 2001. "Automatic Word Processing: A New Forum for Hypnotic Expression." *American Journal of Clinical Hypnosis* 44 (1): 27–36. https://doi.org/10.1080/00029157.2001.10403453.

Anbar, Ran D. 2001. "Self-Hypnosis for Management of Chronic Dyspnea in Pediatric Patients." *Pediatrics* 107 (2): e21. https://doi.org/10.1542/peds.107.2.e21.

Anbar, Ran D. 2001. "The Closure and the Rings: When a Physician Disregards a Patient's Wish." *Pediatric Pulmonology* 31 (1): 76–79.

Anbar, Ran D. 2004. "Stressors Associated with Dyspnea in Childhood: Patients' Insights and a Case Report." *American Journal of Clinical Hypnosis* 47 (2): 93–101. https://doi.org/10.1080/00029157.2004.10403628.

Anbar, Ran D. 2008. "Subconscious Guided Therapy with Hypnosis." *American Journal of Clinical Hypnosis* 50 (4): 323–334. https://doi.org/10.10 80/00029157.2008.10404299.

Anbar, Ran D. 2008. "Treatment of Psychological Complications of Prematurity with Self-Hypnosis: A Case Report." *Clinical Pediatrics* 48 (1): 106–108. https://doi.org/10.1177/0009922808322303.

Anbar, Ran D. 2014. "Hypnosis for Children with Chronic Disease." In William C. Wester and Laurence I. Sugarman (eds.), *Therapeutic Hypnosis with Children and Adolescents* (403–431). 2nd ed. Carmarthen, UK: Crown House Publishing.

Anbar, Ran D., and Howard R. Hall. 2004. "Childhood Habit Cough Treated with Self-Hypnosis." *Journal of Pediatrics* 144 (2): 213–217. https://doi.org/10.1016/j.jpeds.2003.10.041.

Anbar, Ran D., and D. A. Hehir. 2000. "Hypnosis as a Diagnostic Modality for Vocal Cord Dysfunction." *Pediatrics* 106 (6): e81–81. https://doi.org/10.1542/peds.106.6.e81.

Anbar, Ran D., and Julie H. Linden. 2010. "Understanding Dissociation and Insight in the Treatment of Shortness of Breath with Hypnosis: A Case Study." *American Journal of Clinical Hypnosis* 52 (4): 263–273. https://doi.org/10.1080/00029157.2010.10401731.

Anbar, Ran D., and Vaani V. Murthy. 2010. "Reestablishment of Hope as an Intervention for a Patient with Cystic Fibrosis Awaiting Lung Transplantation." *Journal of Alternative and Complementary Medicine* 16 (9): 1007–1010. https://doi.org/10.1089/acm.2010.0107.

Bailey, Lucanne Magill. 1986. "Music Therapy in Pain Management." *Journal of Pain and Symptom Management* 1 (1): 25–28. https://doi.org/10.1016/s0885-3924(86)80024-0.

Barber, Theodore Xenophon, and David Smith Calverley. 1963. "'Hypnotic-Like' Suggestibility in Children and Adults." *Journal of Abnormal and Social Psychology* 66 (6): 589–597. https://doi.org/10.1037/h0041709.

Bargh, John A., and Ezequiel Morsella. 2008. "The Unconscious Mind." *Perspectives on Psychological Science* 3 (1): 73–79. https://doi.org/10.1111/j.1745-6916.2008.00064.x.

Benedetti, Fabrizio, Giuliano Maggi, Leonardo Lopiano, Michele Lanotte, Innocenzo Rainero, Sergio Vighetti, and Antonella Pollo. 2003. "Open Versus Hidden Medical Treatments: The Patient's Knowledge About a Therapy Affects the Therapy Outcome." *Prevention & Treatment* 6 (1), Article 1a. https://doi.org/10.1037/1522-3736.6.1.61a.

Bodde, N. M. G., J. L. Brooks, G. A. Baker, P. A. J. M. Boon, J. G. M. Hendriksen, and A. P. Aldenkamp. 2009. "Psychogenic Non-epileptic Seizures—Diagnostic Issues: A Critical Review." *Clinical Neurology and Neurosurgery* 111 (1): 1–9. https://doi.org/10.1016/j.clineuro.2008.09.028.

Brunet, Alain, Daniel Saumier, Aihua Liu, David L. Streiner, Jacques Tremblay, and Roger K. Pitman. 2018. "Reduction of PTSD Symptoms with Pre-reactivation Propranolol Therapy: A Randomized Controlled Trial." *American Journal of Psychiatry* 175 (5): 427–433. https://doi.org/10.1176/appi.ajp.2017.17050481.

Christopher, Kent L., Raymond P. Wood, R. Christa Eckert, Florence B. Blager, Roy A. Raney, and Joseph F. Souhrada. 1983. "Vocal-Cord Dysfunction Presenting as Asthma." *New England Journal of Medicine* 308 (26): 1566–1570. https://doi.org/10.1056/nejm198306303082605.

Cojan, Yann, Lakshmi Waber, Sophie Schwartz, Laurent Rossier, Alain Forster, and Patrik Vuilleumier. 2009. "The Brain Under Self-Control: Modulation of Inhibitory and Monitoring Cortical Networks During Hypnotic Paralysis." *Neuron* 62 (6): 862–875. https://doi.org/10.1016/j.neuron.2009.05.021.

Dikel, William, and Karen Olness. 1980. "Self-Hypnosis, Biofeedback, and Voluntary Peripheral Temperature Control in Children." *Pediatrics* 66 (3): 335–340.

Elkins, Gary, William Fisher, Aimee Johnson, and Jim Sliwinski. 2012. "Clinical Hypnosis for the Palliative Care of Cancer Patients." *Oncology* 26 (8): 26–30.

Flynn, Niamh. 2018. "Systematic Review of the Effectiveness of Hypnosis for the Management of Headache." *International Journal of Clinical and Experimental Hypnosis* 66 (4): 343–352. https://doi.org/10.1080/00207144.2 018.1494432.

"Free Hypnosis to Be More Creative." Melbourne Hypnotherapy Clinic. https://melbournehypnotherapyclinic.com/free-hypnosis-be-more-creative.

Fretzayas, Andrew, Maria Moustaki, Ioanna Loukou, and Konstantinos Douros. 2017. "Differentiating Vocal Cord Dysfunction from Asthma." *Journal of Asthma and Allergy* 10 (October): 277–283. https://doi.org/ 10.2147/jaa.s146007.

Gilgoff, Rachel, Leena Singh, Kadiatou Koita, Breanna Gentile, and Sara Silverio Marques. 2020. "Adverse Childhood Experiences, Outcomes, and Interventions." *Pediatric Clinics of North America* 67 (2): 259–273. https:// doi.org/10.1016/j.pcl.2019.12.001.

Hammond, D. Corydon. 2007. "Review of the Efficacy of Clinical Hypnosis with Headaches and Migraines." *International Journal of Clinical and Experimental Hypnosis* 55 (2): 207–219. https://doi.org/10.1080/ 00207140601177921.

Heenan, Deirdre. 2006. "Art as Therapy: An Effective Way of Promoting Positive Mental Health?" *Disability & Society* 21 (2): 179–191. https://doi .org/10.1080/09687590500498143.

Hovec, Frank J. Mac. 1975. "Hypnosis Before Mesmer." *American Journal of Clinical Hypnosis* 17 (4): 215–220. https://doi.org/10.1080/00029157.1975 .10403747.

"Hypnotherapy for Highly Creative People." Browning Clinical Hypnotherapy. https://browninghypnotherapy.com/hypnotherapy-for -highly-creative-people-3.

Jacknow, Dale S., Jeanne M. Tschann, Michael P. Link, and W. Thomas Boyce. 1994. "Hypnosis in the Prevention of Chemotherapy-Related Nausea and Vomiting in Children: A Prospective Study." *Journal of Developmental and Behavioral Pediatrics* 15 (4): 258–264. https://doi.org/10.1097/00004703-199408000-00007.

Jardine, David L., Wouter Wieling, Michele Brignole, Jacques W. M. Lenders, Richard Sutton, and Julian Stewart. 2018. "The Pathophysiology of the Vasovagal Response." *Heart Rhythm* 15 (6): 921–929. https://doi.org/10.1016/j.hrthm.2017.12.013.

Jiang, Heidi, Matthew P. White, Michael D. Greicius, Lynn C. Waelde, and David Spiegel. 2017. "Brain Activity and Functional Connectivity Associated with Hypnosis." *Cerebral Cortex* 27 (8): 4083–4093. https://doi.org/10.1093/cercor/bhw220.

Kaptchuk, Ted J., Elizabeth Friedlander, John M. Kelley, M. Norma Sanchez, Efi Kokkotou, Joyce P. Singer, Magda Kowalczykowski, Franklin G. Miller, Irving Kirsch, and Anthony J. Lembo. 2010. "Placebos Without Deception: A Randomized Controlled Trial in Irritable Bowel Syndrome." Edited by Isabelle Boutron. *PLoS ONE* 5 (12): e15591. https://doi.org/10.1371/journal.pone.0015591.

Kemper, Kathi J., and Suzanne C. Danhauer. 2005. "Music as Therapy." *Southern Medical Journal* 98 (3): 282–288. https://doi.org/10.1097/01.smj.0000154773.11986.39.

Kentor, Rachel A., and Julie B. Kaplow. 2020. "Supporting Children and Adolescents Following Parental Bereavement: Guidance for Health-Care Professionals." *The Lancet Child & Adolescent Health* 4 (12): 889–898. https://doi.org/10.1016/s2352-4642(20)30184-x.

Keuthen, Nancy J., Richard L. O'Sullivan, Paige Goodchild, Dayami Rodriguez, Michael A. Jenike, and Lee Baer. 1998. "Retrospective Review of Treatment Outcome for 63 Patients with Trichotillomania." *American Journal of Psychiatry* 155 (4): 560–561. https://doi.org/10.1176/ajp.155.4.560.

Kohen, Daniel P., and Karen Olness. 2011. *Hypnosis and Hypnotherapy with Children*. New York: Routledge.

Kravis, Nathan M. 1988. "James Braid's Psychophysiology: A Turning Point in the History of Dynamic Psychiatry." *American Journal of Psychiatry* 145 (10): 1191–1206.

Lazarus, Jeffrey, and Susan K. Klein. 2006. "Treatment of Tics in Patients with Tourette Syndrome with Self-Hypnosis Training Enhanced with Videotapes." *Journal of Developmental & Behavioral Pediatrics* 27 (5): 444–445. https://doi.org/10.1097/00004703-200610000-00063.

Leeb, R. T., R. H. Bitsko, L. Radhakrishnan, P. Martinez, R. Njai, and K. M. Holland. 2020. "Mental Health–Related Emergency Department Visits Among Children Aged <18 Years During the COVID-19 Pandemic— United States, January 1–October 17, 2020." *CDC Morbidity and Mortality Weekly Report* 69: 1675–1680.

Levine, Jon D., Newton C. Gordon, Richard Smith, and Howard L. Fields. 1981. "Analgesic Responses to Morphine and Placebo in Individuals with Postoperative Pain." *Pain* 10 (3): 379–389. https://doi.org/10.1016/0304-3959(81)90099-3.

Linden, Julie H., Anuj Bhardwaj, and Ran D. Anbar. 2006. "Hypnotically Enhanced Dreaming to Achieve Symptom Reduction: A Case Study of 11 Children and Adolescents." *American Journal of Clinical Hypnosis* 48 (4): 279–289. https://doi.org/10.1080/00029157.2006.10401535.

Lippi, Donatella. 2010. "Music and Medicine." *Journal of Multidisciplinary Healthcare* 137 (August). https://doi.org/10.2147/jmdh.s11378.

Lodge, Jackie, Diana Kim Harte, and Gail Tripp. 1998. "Children's Self-Talk Under Conditions of Mild Anxiety." *Journal of Anxiety Disorders* 12 (2): 153–176. https://doi.org/10.1016/s0887-6185(98)00006-1.

MacPhee, Edward. 2013. "Dissociative Disorders in Medical Settings." *Current Psychiatry Reports* 15 (10). https://doi.org/10.1007/s11920-013-0398-8.

Martínez-Taboas, Alfonso. 2002. "The Role of Hypnosis in the Detection of Psychogenic Seizures." *American Journal of Clinical Hypnosis* 45 (1): 11–20. https://doi.org/10.1080/00029157.2002.10403493.

Mayo Clinic Staff. 2020. "Denial: When It Helps, When It Hurts." Mayo Clinic. April 9. www.mayoclinic.org/healthy-lifestyle/adult-health/in-depth/denial/art-20047926.

Metzger, Frank C. 1947. "Emotions in the Allergic Individual." *American Journal of Psychiatry* 103 (5): 697–699. https://doi.org/10.1176/ajp .103.5.697.

Newberg, Andrew B., and Mark Robert Waldman. 2013. *Words Can Change Your Brain : 12 Conversation Strategies to Build Trust, Resolve Conflict, and Increase Intimacy.* New York: A Plume Book.

Olness, Karen, John Macdonald, and D. L. Uden. 1987. "Comparison of Self-Hypnosis and Propranolol in the Treatment of Juvenile Classic Migraine." *Pediatrics* 79 (4): 593–597.

Olson, Donald M., Neva Howard, and Richard J. Shaw. 2008. "Hypnosis-Provoked Nonepileptic Events in Children." *Epilepsy & Behavior* 12 (3): 456–459. https://doi.org/10.1016/j.yebeh.2007.12.003.

Otgaar, Henry, Mark L. Howe, Lawrence Patihis, Harald Merckelbach, Steven Jay Lynn, Scott O. Lilienfeld, and Elizabeth F. Loftus. 2019. "The Return of the Repressed: The Persistent and Problematic Claims of Long-Forgotten Trauma." *Perspectives on Psychological Science* 14 (6): 1072–1095. https://doi.org/10.1177/1745691619862306.

Palsson, Olafur S. 2015. "Hypnosis Treatment of Gastrointestinal Disorders: A Comprehensive Review of the Empirical Evidence." *American Journal of Clinical Hypnosis* 58 (2): 134–158. https://doi.org/10.1080/00029157.2015 .1039114.

Patterson, David R., John J. Everett, G. Leonard Burns, and Janet A. Marvin. 1992. "Hypnosis for the Treatment of Burn Pain." *Journal of Consulting and Clinical Psychology* 60 (5): 713–717. https://doi.org/10.1037/0022 -006x.60.5.713.

Pickles, Diane M., Stacey L. Lihn, Thomas F. Boat, and Carole Lannon. 2020. "A Roadmap to Emotional Health for Children and Families with Chronic Pediatric Conditions." *Pediatrics* 145 (2) (February): e20191324. https://doi .org/10.1542/peds.2019-1324.

Poulsen, Bruce C., and William J. Matthews. 2003. "Correlates of Imaginative and Hypnotic Suggestibility in Children." *Contemporary Hypnosis* 20 (4): 198–208. https://doi.org/10.1002/ch.278.

Raz, Amir, Theodore Shapiro, Jin Fan, and Michael I. Posner. 2002. "Hypnotic Suggestion and the Modulation of Stroop Interference." *Archives of General Psychiatry* 59 (12): 1155. https://doi.org/10.1001/archpsyc.59.12.1155.

Shenefelt, Philip D. 2011. "Ideomotor Signaling: From Divining Spiritual Messages to Discerning Subconscious Answers During Hypnosis and Hypnoanalysis, a Historical Perspective." *American Journal of Clinical Hypnosis* 53 (3): 157–167. https://doi.org/10.1080/00029157.2011.10401754.

Sher, Heather. 2019. "The Grace of Denial." *New England Journal of Medicine* 380 (2): 118–119. https://doi.org/10.1056/nejmp1810685.

Smith, Helen E., Christina J. Jones, Matthew Hankins, Andy Field, Alice Theadom, Richard Bowskill, Rob Horne, and Anthony J. Frew. 2015. "The Effects of Expressive Writing on Lung Function, Quality of Life, Medication Use, and Symptoms in Adults with Asthma." *Psychosomatic Medicine* 77 (4): 429–437. https://doi.org/10.1097/psy.0000000000000166.

Smyth, Joshua M. 1998. "Written Emotional Expression: Effect Sizes, Outcome Types, and Moderating Variables." *Journal of Consulting and Clinical Psychology* 66 (1): 174–184. https://doi.org/10.1037/0022-006x.66.1.174.

"Sour Mood Getting You Down? Get Back to Nature." 2018. Harvard Health Publishing. July. www.health.harvard.edu/mind-and-mood/sour-mood-getting-you-down-get-back-to-nature.

Stickley, Theodore, Nicola Wright, and Mike Slade. 2018. "The Art of Recovery: Outcomes from Participatory Arts Activities for People Using Mental Health Services." *Journal of Mental Health* 27 (4): 367–373. https://doi.org/10.1080/09638237.2018.1437609.

Stuckey, Heather L., and Jeremy Nobel. 2010. "The Connection Between Art, Healing, and Public Health: A Review of Current Literature." *American*

Journal of Public Health 100 (2): 254–263. https://doi.org/10.2105/ajph
.2008.156497.

Thomson, Linda. 2011. *Harry the Hypno-potamus: Metaphorical Tales for the Treatment of Children.* Carmarthen, UK: Crown House Publishing.

Tillmann, Suzanne, Danielle Tobin, William Avison, and Jason Gilliland. 2018. "Mental Health Benefits of Interactions with Nature in Children and Teenagers: A Systematic Review." *Journal of Epidemiology and Community Health* 72 (10): 958–966. https://doi.org/10.1136/jech-2018-210436.

Trauger-Querry, Barbara, and Katherine Ryan Haghighi. 1999. "Balancing the Focus: Art and Music Therapy for Pain Control and Symptom Management in Hospice Care." *Hospice Journal* 14 (1): 25–38. https://doi .org/10.1080/0742-969x.1999.11882912.

Vermeire, E., H. Hearnshaw, P. Royen, and J. Denekens. "Patient Adherence to Treatment: Three Decades of Research: A Comprehensive Review." *Journal of Clinical Pharmacy and Therapeutics* 26 (2001): 331–342.

Vlieger, Arine M., Carla Menko-Frankenhuis, Simone C. S. Wolfkamp, Ellen Tromp, and Marc A. Benninga. 2007. "Hypnotherapy for Children with Functional Abdominal Pain or Irritable Bowel Syndrome: A Randomized Controlled Trial." *Gastroenterology* 133 (5): 1430–1436. https://doi.org/ 10.1053/j.gastro.2007.08.072.

Wagner, K. D. 2009. "Anxiety Disorders in Children and Adolescents: New Findings." *Psychiatric Times* 32 (3): 483–524.

White, Mathew P., Ian Alcock, James Grellier, Benedict W. Wheeler, Terry Hartig, Sara L. Warber, Angie Bone, Michael H. Depledge, and Lora E. Fleming. 2019. "Spending at Least 120 Minutes a Week in Nature Is Associated with Good Health and Wellbeing." *Scientific Reports* 9 (1). https://doi.org/10.1038/s41598-019-44097-3.

White, Rachel E., and Stephanie M. Carlson. 2015. "What Would Batman Do? Self-Distancing Improves Executive Function in Young Children." *Developmental Science* 19 (3): 419–426. https://doi.org/10.1111/desc .12314.

Yang, Seoyon, and Min Cheol Chang. 2019. "Chronic Pain: Structural and
    Functional Changes in Brain Structures and Associated Negative Affective
    States." *International Journal of Molecular Sciences* 20 (13). https://doi.org/
    10.3390/ijms20133130.

Zhu, Junjia, Muhammad Hussain, Aditya Joshi, Cristina I. Truica, Darya
    Nesterova, Jolene Collins, Erika F. H. Saunders, Michael Hayes, Joseph J.
    Drabick, and Monika Joshi. 2020. "Effect of Creative Writing on Mood
    in Patients with Cancer." *BMJ Supportive & Palliative Care* 10 (1): 64–67.
    doi:10.1136/bmjspcare-2018-001710Zhu.

Index

abdominal pain, management of, 141–43

academic issues, hypnosis and, 101–2

acceptance: and grief, 213; and spirituality, 223–25; and subconscious, 173–85; of whole self, 259–61

action, one positive step, 180; recommendations for, 261–63

acupuncture, 17

adrenaline, 193

advice, subconscious and, 165

advocacy: for hypnosis, 271–72; recommendations for, 247–48

age: imagery and, 77–80; subconscious and, 126–27

age progression, 208

age regression, 207–8

Aidan, and bedtime routine, 234–35

allergies, 11–12, 83, 190, 244

Amy, and cry for help, 177–79

amygdala, 54

anchoring, 67; concrete objects for, 78–79, 86

anger, 29; grief and, 212–13

Aniya, and subconscious, 176

anorexia, 111–12

anxiety, 11, 14, 29, 195–96; and anorexia, 111; and breathing, 36; hypnosis for, 89, 93–102; and nightmares, 156–57; prevalence of, 93; and vasovagal syncope, 103–4

arts, and spirituality, 221

asthma, 7; emotions and, 36; hypnosis for, 23; versus vocal cord dysfunction, 40

attitude: and hypnosis, 45–46, 90; subconscious and, 196

awesome places, focusing on, 227

bedtime routines, 234–35

belief: effectiveness of, 63–64; reasons for, 59–69, 182–83;

recommendations for, 243–44; in
    something bigger, 249–50
Belle (character), 78
Benjamin, and poetry, 148–50
bias, and interpretation, 121, 125
biofeedback, 17
blurring emotions: physical
    symptoms and, 141; subconscious
    and, 128; very young children
    and, 77–78
Braid, James, 25
brain: chronic pain and, 29; hypnotic
    state and, 23–24; seizures and,
    83–84; words and, 54
breathing, 171; and perspective,
    254–55; and relaxation, 15; and
    self-soothing, 246
Bruce, and seizures, 83–88

calm, tips for, 251–65
centering. See under relaxation
CF. See cystic fibrosis
change, wishing for, 223–25
Charlie, and loss, 212–15
child-led interviews: and
    dreams, 154–55, 157–58; and
    empowerment, 132, 191–92; and
    hypnosis instruction, 235–37;
    and imagery, 59, 77, 85–86; and
    intention, 104–6; respect and, 183;
    and subconscious, 119, 124; and
    success of hypnosis, 59
children: and powerlessness, 189;
    and power of words, 54–55; and
    problem definition, 37

Children's Miracle Network, 142, 145
Chloe, and phobia, 204–6
chronic illnesses, 8–10; hypnosis for,
    26; positive words and, 55
coach, inner guide as, 98–100
communication: denial and, 171;
    subconscious and, 123–24
competition, therapy and, 100–101
Connor, and conversion disorder,
    177
conscience, subconscious as, 168
consciousness, levels of, 117
consequences, potential, 184–85
control-center imagery, 77; and
    fever management, 88; and pain
    management, 76
conversion disorders, 176–77
cooperation: and hypnotizability, 24;
    and intention, 104–12
coping tips, 251–65
corpus callosum, 84
cough, 129–38
COVID-19 pandemic, 251–52,
    256–57, 262
creativity: home activities for, 150;
    and spirituality, 221; subconscious
    and, 127, 141–50; and treatment,
    51
creatures: as models, 131, 152;
    mourning, 218; and pain
    evaluation, 75
crises, tips for, 251–65
Cristobal, and pandemic, 256–57
cystic fibrosis (CF), 7, 8–10, 156,
    192–93

About the Author

Ran D. Anbar, MD, FAAP, is board certified in both pediatric pulmonology and general pediatrics, offering hypnosis and counseling services at Center Point Medicine in La Jolla, California, and Syracuse, New York. Dr. Anbar is also past president, fellow, and approved consultant of the American Society of Clinical Hypnosis.

Dr. Anbar launched CPM Franchise Group in 2021, which recruits pediatricians to learn how to use hypnosis and open Center Point Medicine practices around the country.

Dr. Anbar is a leader in clinical hypnosis. His twenty-four years of experience have allowed him to successfully treat over seven thousand children with hypnosis and counseling. He also served as a professor of pediatrics and medicine and the director of pediatric pulmonology at SUNY Upstate Medical University in Syracuse, New York, for twenty-one years.

Dr. Anbar has worked as a guest editor and advisory editor for the *American Journal of Clinical Hypnosis*. His experience has offered him the opportunity to direct and codirect more than twenty clinic workshops on the subject of pediatric hypnosis. He has also trained more than a thousand health care providers and lectured all over the world.

In addition to his teaching and lecturing experiences, Dr. Anbar has been the principal investigator in ten published case studies of pediatric hypnosis and involved in more than fifty other research trials of children with cystic fibrosis and other pulmonary disorders. He is a published author of more than fifty articles, abstracts, and book chapters on pediatric functional disorders and pediatric hypnosis.

Graduating from the University of California, San Diego, with undergraduate degrees in biology and psychology, Dr. Anbar earned his medical degree from the University of Chicago Pritzker School of Medicine. He completed his pediatric residency and pediatric pulmonary fellowship training at the Massachusetts General Hospital and Harvard Medical School in Boston. Dr. Anbar received training in hypnosis from the Society of Developmental and Behavioral Pediatrics and the American Society of Clinical Hypnosis.

Website: centerpointhypnosis.com